PEDIATRIC CANCER SURVIVORS

Edited by **Karen Wonders**
and **Brittany Stout**

Pediatric Cancer Survivors
http://dx.doi.org/10.5772/63327
Edited by Karen Wonders and Brittany Stout

Contributors

Orsolya Németh, Jake Kleinmahon, Bruce Landeck, Ayşe Gürol, Sevinç Polat, Christopher Kuo, Paul Kent, Nupur Mittal, Karen Wonders

Published by InTech
Janeza Trdine 9, 51000 Rijeka, Croatia

Publishing Process Manager Ana Simcic
Technical Editor SPi Global
Cover InTech Design team

First published June, 2017
Printed in Croatia
Legal deposit, Croatia: National and University Library in Zagreb

Additional hard copies can be obtained from orders@intechopen.com

Pediatric Cancer Survivors, Edited by Karen Wonders and Brittany Stout
p. cm.
Print ISBN 978-953-51-3219-6
Online ISBN 978-953-51-3220-2

For EU product safety concerns:
IN TECH d.o.o., Prolaz Marije Krucifikse Kozulić 3, 51000 Rijeka, Croatia,
info@intechopen.com or visit our website at intechopen.com.

Meet the editor

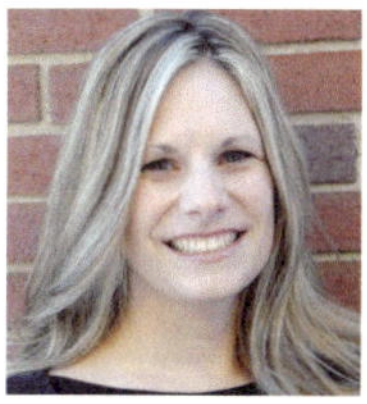

Editor, Karen Wonders, PhD, FACSM, is the founder and director of Maple Tree Cancer Alliance, a nonprofit organization that provides free exercise training, nutrition counseling, and spiritual support to individuals battling cancer. She also works as a professor of Exercise Science at Wright State University and is the program director of the Sports Science Program. Dr. Wonders is an active speaker who has given over 100 presentations on the national, state, and local levels as well as authored several peer-reviewed manuscripts, books, and book chapters on healthy living in cancer recovery. She serves more than 2,500 patients every year in Maple Tree's three offices and thousands of participants in her online fitness programs. Dr. Wonders lives in Dayton, Ohio, with her husband Andrew and their seven children.

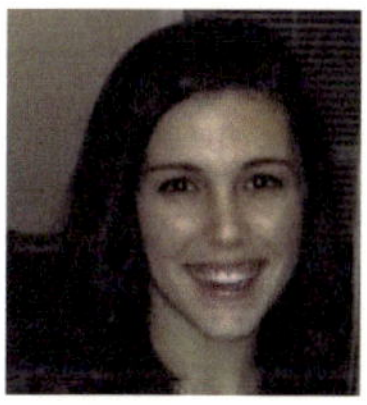

Co-Editor, Brittany Stout is the research coordinator for Maple Tree Cancer Alliance. She has been with the organization for about 3 years, focusing her first year on exercise training and transitioning to more research-based projects recently. She obtained her undergraduate degree in Exercise Science at the University of Toledo, graduating in 2013. From there, she went on to study at the University of Dayton, achieving her master's degree in Exercise Science as well. While at the University of Dayton, she collaborated with Maple Tree Cancer Alliance to complete her thesis on the feasibility of online exercise and nutrition programs for child cancer survivors. She hopes to continue her work with cancer survivors, publishing research, and furthering knowledge in the field.

Contents

Preface

Due to advancements in health technology and the treatment of cancer, the number of cancer survivors in the USA has increased significantly in recent years. Even though the amount of cancer survivors has substantially increased, the quality of life of these individuals tends to remain diminished. Many of these survivors continue to struggle with impaired physical and mental health, spanning from months to years after completion of treatments. These can include depressed cardiopulmonary function, fatigue, decreased muscle strength, and altered physical function. Emotionally, patients often experience depression, slow information processing, difficulty understanding, and impaired judgment. Damages to mental health have been reported to lead to issues affecting nutrition including decreased appetite and alterations in taste and smell. The combined impairments can all negatively affect and diminish a cancer survivors' health-related quality of life.

When a child develops cancer, it presents a host of unique challenges. Cancer develops in 1 to 500 children. Typically, the type of cancers that develop in children is different than those that develop in adults, in that they are often the result of a DNA mutation rather than environmental or lifestyle risk factors. Leukemia, brain and central nervous system tumors, and neuroblastomas are the most common cancer types in child populations. Children tend to respond better to anticancer treatments, including chemotherapy and radiation. However, long-term side effects are common in children, often requiring follow-up care and lifestyle intervention for the rest of their lives. The percentage of 5-year survivors was over 50% for the most common cancers. This suggests that a majority of cancers in this population are highly survivable. As such, research should focus on aspects of recovery and survivorship for these individuals. This book will explore issues related to pediatric cancer and their associated treatments.

Karen Wonders Ph.D., FACSM
Program Director, Sports Science Professor
Department of Kinesiology and Health
Wright State University, United States

Brittany Stout, MS
Clinical Research Coordinator
Maple Tree Cancer Alliance

Chapter 1

Introductory Chapter: Pediatric Cancer Survivors

Karen Wonders and Brittany Stout

Additional information is available at the end of the chapter

http://dx.doi.org/10.5772/intechopen.69147

1. Introduction

Receiving a cancer diagnosis is very disheartening, but hearing a diagnosis for a child takes on a whole new set of knowledge and emotions. Pediatric cancers (ages 0–19) are a rare and challenging time for families, as well as for pediatricians and oncologists. While cancer is much less common among children compared to adults, 1 in 285 children will be diagnosed with the disease before the age of 20 years in the United States [2]. The incidence rate of pediatric cancers in the United States has increased slightly over the years (0.6% per year [2]), but rates of a 5-year survival for many of these cancer types have increased to an even greater degree due to advances in modern technology. For most cases, the cause of a childhood cancer is inconclusive, and gathering sound data in the area is challenging because pediatric cancers are so rare. From what researchers have been able to gather, there have been links between certain gene mutations passed from mother to child as well as an increased risk in children who experience gene changes during early growth in the womb [1].

There is a slight variability in pediatric characteristics relating to incidence rates and survival. These differences can be seen in sex, ethnicity, and age, but the reasons behind these variances are not well understood. While the rates of 5-year survivors are similar, incidence and mortality rates tend to be lower in girls than in boys. Conversely, in adolescents, incidence rates are similar and girls have lower mortality rates compared to boys [2]. There is even more variability when looking at ethnic background. Caucasian and Hispanic children have the highest incidence rates for developing cancer compared to African American children who have the lowest incidents rates but experience the lowest survival rates as well [3]. Children with Down syndrome are also at an increased risk of developing leukemia [1].

2. Differences in pediatric and adult cancers

Types of cancers that develop in child and adolescent populations differ from the adult population in several ways. The most prevalent types of cancers seen in children are leukemia (26%), cancers of the brain and central nervous systems (18%), and lymphoma (14%) [4]. These cancers are typically only seen in child populations, and this is due to the embryonic or developmental nature of the cancer origin. Since these cancers develop either while in-utero or develop from embryonic tissue, these cancers are rarely seen in adult populations. Those diagnosed closer to adolescence tend to reflect similar cancers to that of the adult population. Pediatric cancers are often the result of DNA mutations that happen very early in life (sometimes even before birth) and are not strongly linked to lifestyle or environmental cancers the way adult populations are [5].

Treatment mechanisms also differ in pediatric and adult populations. Some treatments given to adults are deemed unsafe for children due to their destructive nature [1]. Many times, pediatric cancers are handled with a team of experts, or the child's oncology group (COG), in order to determine the best routes of health care [1].

3. Types of childhood cancers

Pediatric cancers represent 1% of all new cancer cases, but these cancers are usually fast developing and require multidisciplinary teams including pediatric oncologists, surgeons, radiation oncologists, and other specialists [5]. Cancers in the pediatric populations can be further divided into common types of cancer affecting children (ages 0–14) and adolescents (ages 15–19). The most common cancer types for children are lymphocytic leukemia, brain and central nervous system, neuroblastoma, and non-Hodgkin's lymphoma, while adolescents are more commonly diagnosed with Hodgkin's lymphoma and thyroid carcinoma [2, 5].

Similar to adult populations, pediatric cancer treatments come accompanied with many harsh side effects. Milder side effects can include rash, pain, and upset stomach and can usually be eased with medication and healthy living [1]. Cancer can affect these children very early in life, sometimes interrupting the natural growth and development processes. Harsher side effects experienced with treatment can interrupt or halt the natural development in organs and tissues, changing their function [1, 5].

4. Prevention, treatment, and outcomes

Obtaining sound data in terms of prevention has been found to be difficult as pediatric cancers are so rare, and many prevention mechanisms would be attributed to womb development. What is known regarding prevention is that there is a lack of control in terms of reducing the risk of incidence. Research has shown that physical activity and proper nutrition (to name a

http://dx.doi.org/10.5772/intechopen.69147

few) can improve treatment and survivorship parameters, but there has been little progress in terms of prevention [6].

For most cancer types in the pediatric community, the treatment option that tends to respond best is chemotherapy. Children are often able to handle higher doses of chemo drugs for shorter periods of time [1]. In addition, children's bodies are better capable of handling chemotherapy treatments than adults. Radiation treatment is also an option for pediatric cancers, but children (especially very young children) are more likely to be affected negatively, and radiation therapy can lead to potential long-term side effects that can be experienced later in life. As pediatric cancers affect children at a young age, along with there being an increase in survivors, management and frequent follow-up care are important.

5. Conclusion

Within the content of the following chapters, these topics and points will be discussed in more detail. The information found within this book will enhance professionals' knowledge in the field of pediatric oncology and provide a sounder outlook for incidence, prevention, treatment, and outcomes. Although further research needs to be done in this area for more specific knowledge to be gained, this book is filled with the most up-to-date information in the field of pediatric oncology thus far.

Author details

Karen Wonders[1]* and Brittany Stout[2]

*Address all correspondence to: karen.wonders@wright.edu

1 Department of Kinesiology and Health, Wright State University, Dayton, USA

2 Maple Tree Cancer Alliance, Dayton, USA

References

[1] ADAM. How Childhood Cancers are Different from Adult Cancers. 2016. Available from: https://medlineplus.gov/ency/patientinstructions/000845.htm

[2] American Cancer Society. Cancer Facts & Figures. Special Section: Cancer in Children and Adolescence. 2014. Available from https://www.cancer.org/content/dam/cancer-org/research/cancer-facts-and-statistics/annual-cancer-facts-and-figures/2014/special-section-cancer-in-children-and-adolescents-cancer-facts-and-figures-2014.pdf

[3] National Cancer Institute. Childhood Cancers: Cancer in Children and Adolescents. 2014. Available from www.cancer.gov/types/childhood-cancers/child-adolescent-cancers-fact-sheet

[4] Ward E, DeSantis C, Robbins A, Kohler B, Jemal A. Childhood and adolescent cancer statistics, 2014. CA: A Cancer Journal for Clinicians. 2014;**64**:83–103. DOI: 10.3322/caac.21219

[5] American Cancer Society. What are the Differences between Cancers in Adults and Children? 2016. Available from https://www.cancer.org/cancer/cancer-in-children/differences-adults-children.html

[6] Yelton L, Forbis S. Influences and barriers on physical activity in pediatric oncology patients. Frontiers in Pediatrics. 2016;**4**:1–9. DOI: 10.3389/fped.2016.00131

Chapter 2

Dental and Craniofacial Effects on Childhood Cancer Survivors

Orsolya Németh

Additional information is available at the end of the chapter

http://dx.doi.org/10.5772/67040

Abstract

The availability and adoption of modern therapeutic protocols for childhood cancer have continuously reduced the mortality rate of childhood malignancies in most countries over the past decades. Children being treated for cancer are actively growing, creating unique problems not only in the short-term but also in the long-term development of both the orofacial hard and soft tissue. Complications during and after cancer therapy depend on the type of malignancy, age at diagnosis, and the drugs used during the therapy. The adverse oral effects of irradiation have long been known, and high-dose chemotherapy can cause similar oral late effects, such as dental disturbances, delayed tooth eruption, oral mucosa changes, and craniofacial effects. There are many protocols to prevent acute oral toxicity and infections like mucositis, candidiasis, or hyposalivation. The aim of this chapter is to define the short-term and long-term effects of cancer therapy on the oral health.

Keywords: oral health, dental disturbances, craniofacial effects, saliva flow rate

1. Introduction

1.1. Craniofacial development

An understanding of dental and craniofacial effects of cancer therapy is an essential knowledge of distinct mechanism of postnatal craniofacial development, growth, and capacities for adaptation during growth.

The craniofacial complex can be organized according to four anatomic regions: desmocranium, chondrocranium, splanchnocranium, and the most specialized anatomic component, dentition.

There are three principal growth-related cranial base synchondroses that separate the bones of cranial base at birth. Fuses of intersphenoid synchondrosis finished around the time of birth and it does not contribute to postnatal growth. The sphenoethmoidal synchondrosis is most active with respect to growth of the cranial base through approximately 7 years of age (synchondrosis loses its cartilage phenotype). Growth of the anterior cranial base is essentially complete. As a result, the anterior wall of sella turcica, the greater wing of the sphenoid, and the cribriform plate are commonly used after age 7 as stable reference structures for analyses of lateral cephalograms. The third synchondrosis (sphenooccipital) is most prominent throughout the period of active craniofacial growth and fuses only after puberty at 16–19 years.

The cranial base undergoes a dramatic shift in its growth pattern during the early postnatal years. Cranial base dimensions (anterior and posterior lengths) and cranial base angulations show greater growth changes at the age of 2 and 3 years. The changes after 2–3 years of age are smaller and steady. So the irradiation in this time causes the greatest cranial disturbances.

The midface at the time of birth is well developed, but slightly relative to the neurocranium. Significant anterior and vertical growth of the midface through the first several years after birth can be observed due to interstitial cartilaginous growth of midline nasal septum. Nasomaxillary complex of postnatal development occurs via intramembranous ossification except nasal septum. Growth at the sutures of midface leads to inferior and anterior, and lateral midfacial displacements means vertical, transverse, and anteroposterior changes. Growth continues until premaxillary/maxillary suture closes at 3–5 years of life [1]. The major intermaxillary growth sites are midpalatal and transpalatal sutures, associated with transverse and anteroposterior midface growth. Growth of midpalatal and transpalatal sutures continues until 20–25 years of age [2, 3]. The midface undergoes a complex remodeling pattern throughout childhood and adolescence. The length of entire maxilla and dental arches, and height of the midface are increased by continued development of the dentition and alveolar bone. Growth of cranial base displaces the maxilla in a downward and forward direction [4]. The age of 7 years is something of a benchmark for growth of the midface [4]. Relatively, anterior cranial base is stable but the growth of cartilages of the nasal capsule and nasal septum changes significantly. The cartilaginous nasal capsule becomes ossified and the nasal septum, which remains cartilaginous throughout life, decreases significantly in growth activity. Structures within the midfacial complex also affect its displacement and rotation. Growth of the eyeball is associated with both the anterior and lateral displacements of the midface; enucleation of the eyeball during growth results in deficiencies in the anterior and lateral growth of the midface [5]. Sexual dimorphism increases substantially throughout the midfacial complex. Adult males are larger and wider midfaces than females. The reason is males have the two extra years of childhood's growth; males enter the adolescence phase of growth at 12 years of age, while females enter at 10 years.

During postnatal development, mandible increases in size as a result of the combined processes of proliferation and ossification of secondary cartilage at the condyle, as well as differential formation and remodeling of bone along the entire surface of the mandible. Because the posterior mandible generally undergoes greater inferior displacement than the anterior mandible, the mandible rotates forward. Growth of the mandible is expressed in a downward and forward growth direction relative to the rest of the cranium. In this overall pattern, the growth of the mandible follows the growth of the midface. As the midface is translated downward and forward, the mandible keeps pace in the normally growing face [4, 6]. Midfacial growth and the associated changes in the position of the maxillary dentition are also thought to play an important role in mandibular growth displacements [7–9].

1.2. Dental development

The primary (milk teeth) and secondary dentitions all form in essentially the same manner, although at different times. The entire primary dentition is initiated between 6th and 8th week in utero, the successional permanent teeth between the 20th week of embryonic development and 21 years of age for third molar [10]. Teeth development (initiation) is regulated by epithelial-mesenchymal interactions between oral epithelium and neural crest-derived mesenchyme [11]. During the proliferation stage, tooth formation proceeds through increased mitotic activity, leading to the development of ameloblasts and odontoblasts, which produce enamel prism and dentin. The internal enamel rods will differentiate into ameloblasts and then begin the production of enamel rods. During histodifferentiation stage, the cells lose the ability to multiply. Aberrations in initiation and proliferation typically result in failure of tooth development, while insults during histodifferentiation result lead to abnormal structure of enamel and dentin (amelogenesis and dentinogenesis imperfecta, and discolored enamel). Disturbances during morphodifferentiation can cause abnormal shape and size of teeth. The next stage of individual tooth development is appositional growth, while the ameloblast and odontoblast produce a deposition of an extracellular (organic) matrix. The process of mineralization begins with formation of small nidus (ionic calcium and phosphate precipitation), and this nidus increases in size and leads to homogeneously mineralized layer. Environmental insults during due to lack of fusion of the calcospherites, which could leads to less resistant to dental caries.

Root formation begins when the epithelial layers penetrate into underlying mesenchyme and form the Hertwig's epithelial root sheath. This sheath grows around the dental papilla until it encloses the apical foramen. As a result root disturbance, which is a lack of root structure, leads to shortened and tapered root. Root development plays a dominant role in the eruption [6].

2. Short-term effects

Radiotherapy

Radiation therapy of children with malignancies requires attention to physical and biological principles to maximize efficacy and reduce late effects. Biologically, effective forms of radiation produce energetic charged particles in tissue, resulting in direct and indirect ionization of intracellular molecules with attendant biological effect [12]. The reaction of normal tissues to irradiation can occur during or immediately after therapy as acute effects, within 3–6 months after treatment as subacute effects, and later 6 months after radiotherapy as late effects [13].

Acute radiation injury is expressed in rapidly proliferating tissues like mucous membrane. Acute changes follow depletion of the actively proliferating stem cells, time of onset, and degree depending on the size of the stem cell compartment and response of the cell renewal system. Acute effects do not correlate with subacute and late parenchymal complications after radiotherapy [14] (**Table 1**).

Immediate radiation reaction often occurs xerostomia, which is symptomatically expressed within several days of treatment encompassing the salivary glands. The radiotherapy damage to the salivary glands is due to an alteration in their vascular supply.

Chemotherapy

- Oral mucositis and stomatitis
- Xerostomia
- Infections:
    - Bacterial
    - Viral (herpes simplex, varicella zoster, and cytomegalovirus)
    - Fungal (Candida albicans)
- Bleeding: anywhere in the mouth, spontaneous or induced
- Neurotoxicity: bilateral mimics toothache

Radiation therapy

- Oral mucositis and stomatitis
- Xerostomia
- Radiation caries
- Taste alteration
- Infections:
    - Bacterial
    - Viral (herpes simplex, varicella zoster, cytomegalovirus)
    - Fungal (Candida albicans)
- Trismus: inability to open mouth completely osteoradionecrosis

Hematopoietic cell transplantation (HCT)

- Oral mucositis (10–14 days posttransplant)
- Gingival hyperplasia
- Xerostomia
- Viral and fungal infections

Table 1. Short-term effects of cancer therapy in CCS.

Saliva can become sparse, thick, and ropy after just 4–5 fractions [15]. According to Epstein et al. whole stimulated and resting saliva productions are decreased by 36.67 and 47.9%, respectively, by the end of 1 week of RT [16]. The pH after radiation falls from 7.0 to 5.0, which is cariogenic [17, 18]. As the pH and buffering capacity of saliva are low, the minerals of enamel and dentin dissolve easily [19]. Thus, the process of remineralization of the dental hard tissue does not occur in the oral environment of HNC patients after radiotherapy is prone to demineralization. Consequently, remineralization capacity of saliva is hampered [19]. Accompanied by the reduced oral clearance, these effects result in troublesome changes of the oral flora, with an increase in acidogenic and cariogenic microorganisms (*Streptococcus mutans*, *Lactobacillus*, and *Candida* species) [20].

In Spinger's study, it is said that irradiation is thought to have a direct destructive effect on dental hard tissue, especially at the dentinoenamel junction (DEJ) [21].

Chemotherapy

In therapeutic doses, actively dividing normal host tissues, such as mucosal epithelial and bone marrow cells, are sensitive to the cytotoxic effects of anticancer drugs [22]. Unfortunately, the nonselective mechanism of action and resulting low therapeutic indices of these agents mean that high incidence of potentially severe toxicities must be tolerated to administer effective doses [23]. The dose intensity of anticancer drugs is limited primarily. Many drugs have unique toxicities affecting various organs or tissues such as oral complications associated antimetabolites, alkylating agents, plant alkaloids, and antitumor antibiotics [24]. Therapy affects the oral epithelial cell directly by interfering with actual cell production, maturation, and replacement indirectly to bone marrow depression. Myelosuppression (neutropenia and thrombocytopenia) increases risk of mucosal bleeding and viral, bacterial, and fungal oral infection. The most frequented acute complication of methotrexate in mouth is oral intestinal mucositis. Mucositis occur 5–14 days after dose [25–29]. The development of mucositis is related to the concentration of drug (mg/m^2/week) and during exposure [30] (**Table 1**).

Chemotherapy not only affects the rapidly dividing oral mucosa but also alters the volume of saliva, microbial flora, and shelter line of the mucosa. The oral mucosa of these children have a greater mitotic index, so, its complications in children occur more frequently than those in adult patients. Clinical features include swelling, bleeding, dry mouth, desquamation of gingiva and palate, and cracked and dry lips.

HSCT

Stem cell transplantation is the most dramatic example of rescue approach. Children with malignancies are treated with lethal doses of myelosuppressive drugs or combination with total body irradiation and then we expect infusion of stem cell, bone marrow to prevent permanent marrow aplasia. The oral complications of HSCT are xerostomia, mucositis, oral infection, and gingival hyperplasia [31] (**Table 1**).

2.1. Infections (oral mucositis)

The gastrointestinal system's mucosal toxicity is a frequent immediate or short-term side effect of chemotherapy. It appears only when pen torch erythema illuminates the oral cavity, causing extraordinarily severe pain, and thus becoming impossible for the children to eat or drink. In the case of combined therapy, induced mucositis can develop, which can lead to bleeding and infections [32].

The most frequented causes are therapy of 5-FU, azathioprine, bleomycin, cyclophosphamide, dactinomycin, daunorubicin, doxorubicin, nitrogén mustards, melphalan, 6-mercaptopurine, methotrexate, mitomycins-C, novantrone, mithramycin, procarbazine, streptozotocin, 6-thioguanine, and vinblastine [15, 33].

Mucositis or stomatitis occurs due to the damage and destruction of epithelial cells. In principle cancer therapy can be directly impaired by the cell maturation and replacement and leads to bone marrow depression- myelosuppression and immunsuppression (neutropenia, thrombocytopenia) increase the viral (herpes simplex, varicella zoster, cytomegalovirus), bacterial and fungal (Candida albicans) infections or bleeding [25, 27–29].

In the histological aspect, collagen degradation, hyperplasia, glandular degeneration, and dysplasia can be observed. This means that the chemical and microbiological barrier function of mucosal cease and cause reduced humoral factors (antibody and antimicrobial proteins) formation and the agents cause infections.

Management involves maintenance of meticulous oral hygiene, prevention of infection, and maintenance of oral function (swallowing and chewing). Systematic analgetics, ice packs to throat and cheeks 4–6 times daily for 15–20 minutes. Chlorhexidine mouthwashes are not recommended for cytotoxic-induced mucositis [34]. The newest treatment of mucositis can be cryotherapy [35].

2.2. Salivary glands—hyposalivation and xerostomia

The salivary glands derive their fluid with electrolytes, small organic molecules, and macromolecules. Secretion occurs in response to nervous stimulation. Interference with the supply of blood to the gland may lead to decrease in the production of saliva [31, 36, 37]. The secretory cells, the blood supply, and the nerves may all be affected by ionizing radiations. Serous cells are more sensitive to the radiation than the mucous secreting cells. After radiotherapy, the produced saliva is in reduced amount and thicker. Initially, saliva becomes more viscous and lubrication is decreased, as the salivary gland damage progresses. The lips become dry and cracked, and swallowing (dysphagia) and chewing become difficult with pain [38, 39].

The hyposalivation was regarded as a short-term side effect for quite a long-term. In the case of patients undergoing radiotherapy, especially in the area of head and neck irradiation (rare in children), immediate organ toxicity has been described, which could last there for a long time; the patients felt improvement just after 4–12 months [40]. According to Nemeth et al. study, one can draw the conclusion that hyposalivation can be regarded as a long-term side effect after only chemotherapy. Even if this low secretion improves under or after the direct treatment improved a bit, it never ever reaches the pretreatment state [41].

Unstimulated and stimulated saliva flow rate after cancer therapy (radiotherapy and chemotherapy) shows decreasing values. It seems the minor salivary glands constantly try to compensate an appropriate amount of saliva. Nemeth et al. believe that the slight damage in the major salivary glands caused in these children by the chemotherapy was not a real reason for this, since it was compensated by the minor salivary gland function and that is the reason why unstimulated whole saliva flow rate was normal and the buffer capacity of the saliva was higher than in the healthy controls [41].

Lee et al. investigated patients suffering from xerostomia and concluded that the palatal salivary secretion remains held. The palatal minor salivary glands play a protection function in the oral cavity saliva balance with their operation after chemotherapy [42, 43].

Management involves non–alcohol-based mouth rinses, saliva substitute, methyl cellulose, frequent intake of water, and neutral sodium fluoride application [44].

2.3. Herpes virus

Herpes simplex manifests labial and oropharyngitis which may lead to generalized sepsis. Clinically, the lesions appear as clear vesicle eruptions in cluster on the erythematous base, but herpesvirus infection can occur as nondescript and atypical appearance.

Herpes simplex and Herpes zoster infections are acute effects, but when immunosuppression is protracted, persistent infection can occur as indolent ulcers [45–48].

Management includes prevention and treatment with oral or intravenous acyclovir. Oral acyclovir needs large doses because 20–30% of drug is absorbed (750 mg/m^2 per day given every 8 h) [45–48].

2.4. Candida

The most common mucosal infection is thrush, a superficial infection due to Candida albicans. Clinically, the lesions appear as whitish plaques with indurated borders.

Careful attention should be paid to oral hygiene. Clotrimazole troches, nystatin suspension, and oral fluconazole are used to treat the infection (50–100 mg per day) [45, 46].

2.5. Dental caries and periodontal status

Because of the hyposalivation that is an acute side effect of cytostatic agents, children often consume sugary and carbonated soft drinks. As a result of this, the pH of saliva is in the acidic range for long periods because of the qualitative and quantitative changes in the mouth. Because of the oral ulceration, mucositis, and xerostomia during the treatment, the consumption of solid foods may be painful for the children who prefer the soft and mushy foods.

The tooth brushing frequency unfortunately reduces and the duration becomes shorter. These bad habits may persist later and increase late side effects. In most of the study for DMF-T index, the children had mixed so we do not get a valid value. In Dens's examination, the children were 2–17 years old; in Alberth's study they were 4–25 years old, while in Welbury et al., the oral hygiene and periodontal status of survivors of malignant cancer were between 3 and 20 years of age [49–53].

Pajari et al. and Sonis et al. measured DMF-T index, dental hygiene, and gingival index of children with ALL treated. They found the caries' frequency much higher and prevalence of gingivitis is more frequent in the survivor children's group than in the healthy ones' [54–56].

Ayanoglou et al. found gingival overgrowth in rats gum after cyclosporin A injection [57].

Saliva flow seems to play an important role in the rate of dental caries in this population, since saliva has a significant protective effect against cariogenic bacteria due to its enzymatic and immunological activity. The increased caries risk is correlated with the decreased saliva flow rate and the adverse side effect of the treatment can be hyposalivation and concomitant changes of oral microflora.

When teeth are located in the irradiation field, hypovascularity results in a decrease in the circulation through pulpal tissue and increase of the collagen cross-links hydroxylysylpyridinoline and lysylpyridinoline [21]. The effect of radiation on vascular flow to the dentition as a whole also plays a role in this multifaceted caries-promoting cycle [58]. Caries is the main factor contributing to the atypical and comparatively rapid progress of irradiation caries, which may not be explained by hyposalivation alone [16, 59–69]. The increased stiffness is hypothesized due to a radiation-induced decrease in the protein content, with a much greater reduction in the enamel sites as compared to dentin. These changes of mechanical properties and chemical composition can contribute to DEJ biomechanical failure and enamel delamination [Reed]. It was observed that minimal tooth damage occurs below 30 Gy; there was a 2–3 times increased risk of tooth breakdown between 30 and 60 Gy likely related to salivary gland impact; and a more increased risk of tooth damage when the tooth-level dose is above 60 Gy indicating radiation-induced damage to the tooth in addition to salivary gland damage. These findings suggest a direct effect of radiation on tooth structure with increasing radiation dose to the tooth [70–75]. Thus, radiogenic dental damage is the result of reduced salivary flow, as well as possible direct radiogenic damage [76].

Management: try to avoid cariogenic foods and drinks. Perform routine daily personal oral care including biofilm removal and fluoride application (gel and rinse). Dental check up is useful every 3 months.

3. Late effects

Radiotherapy

Late consequences of children cancer can be anticipated based on exposures, but the magnitude of risk and the manifestations in an individual patient are influenced by numerous factors (**Table 2**). There are total dose, fraction size, organ or tissue volume, and type of machine energy in radiotherapy. The extent of oral late effects is dependent upon the age of the children, at the time of treatment.

The lack of specificity of radiotherapy in terms of differentiating neoplastic cells from metabolic active cells may result in dental and craniofacial abnormality. This is a direct effect of

Chemotherapy
• Hyposalivation
• Craniofacial effects
• Orodental disturbances
    • Tooth agenesis
    • Microdontia
    • Enlarged pulp chamber (taurodontism)
    • Enamel hypoplasia (hypomineralization)
    • Enamel discoloration
    • Short, tapered, and blunted roots

Radiation therapy
• Taste alteration
• Xerostomia
• Radiationcaries
• Osteoradionecrosis
• Muscular trismus
• Orodental disturbances
    • Tooth agenesis
    • Microdontia
    • Enlarged pulp chamber (taurodontism)
    • Enamel hypoplasia (hypomineralization)
    • Enamel discoloration
    • Short, tapered, and blunted roots
• Craniofacial effects

Hematopoietic cell transplantation (HCT) • Xerostomia (respond pilocarpine injection) • Nongingival soft tissue growth (like pyogenic granuloma) • Exophytic soft tissue lesion • Gingival hyperplasia • Mucosal lichenoid changes • Mucocele

Table 2. Late-term effects of cancer therapy in CCS.

therapy on growing cells. Indirect effects of therapy may occur in altered hypothalamic-pituitary function resulting in diminished growth hormone production [7–11].

Hard tissue development of craniofacial region occurs with intramembranous and endochondral bone formation and odontogenesis, and the adjoining soft tissue influences hard tissue development. Radiation level of 200cGy in the patient under 6 years of age may be observed with microscopic changes, and when a radiation is greater than 1800 cGy, it affects the calvaria growth and growth in the anteroposterior length. Anomalies of cranial base and orbital development result in a lack of midface development. Enucleation and orbital radiotherapy in growing child age can inhibit the growth of bony structure and detrimental to facial growth especially on transverse facial development. Denys et al. said children with retinoblastoma treated with 3000 cGy are at high risk of craniofacial deformities. Sonis et al. studied craniofacial abnormalities as measured by cephalometric analysis and observed significant deficient mandibular development in 2400 cGy RT before 5 years of age group. Studies of mandibular growth suggest irradiation must exceed 1800 cGy before it is detectable clinically.

Kaste and Hopkins describe a patient with maxillary hypoplasia after 10 years of therapy.

Do not forget craniofacial growth which is not proportional. While calvarial growth is almost completed by age 5 years, the nasomaxillary complex and mandible continue to grow throughout adolescence explaining the huge differences in facial appearance of the 1 and 18 years of age. Most studies may suggest that after 12 years of age radiation-induced facial growth alterations are negligible [77–81].

Growth of alveolar bone is completely dependent on the presence, eruption, and root length of teeth. Odontoblasts are most susceptible to low-dose radiation just prior to their initiation of dentin matrix formation, because presecretory odontoblasts are rapidly proliferating. Following radiotherapy, odontoblastic mitotic activity ceases. Defective enamel is created, because osteodentin interferes with the normal interaction of dentin and enamel. Enamel and dentin defects lead to tooth dwarfism, blunted and tapered root, incomplete calcification, premature apical closure, and lack of eruption [77, 78, 82–87].

Chemotherapy

The late effects of only chemotherapy on the dental- and craniofacial development are limited but some studies of the last 10 years have been shown to affect facial growth directly in humans **Table 2**.

Two chemotherapeutic agents, methotrexate and ifosfamide are well known in the protocols. Both of them are well-known and documented about the negative impact on the growth of bone system. The folic acid antagonist methotrexate can be found in most of the protocols against leukemia and osteosarcoma. Methotrexate over the activity of osteoblasts and osteoclasts decrease the activity of the increasing negative effect on the bone volume and shape. Stanisavljevic and Babcock repeatedly documented osteoporosis and various fractures among children treated against leukemia [88]. Not only after the long-term treatment with MTX, but among the osteosarcoma patients treated with high-dose methotrexate of short-term therapy, Ecklund et al. showed similar lesions in 1997 [89].

After cyclophosphamide analogue ifosfamide treatment, Fanconi syndrome were described several times, which may lead to irreversible impairment of the kidney (hypocalcemia and hypophosphatemia) in the isotretinoin treatment of neuroblastoma, which describes diffuse cortical hyperostosis, ligaments calcification, and periostitis as side effects [90].

Reade and Roberts had already described the cyclophosphamide's negative impact on the development of the rat's incisor in 1978 [91]. Burn Murdoch also mentioned the negative effect of cyclophosphamide [92]. Mataki et al. demonstrated the inhibition of dentinogenesis in the case of vinblastine and colchicine-treated rats [93]. Animal studies have shown that the chemotherapeutic drugs induce qualitative and quantitative changes in the dental tissue, and inhibit the tooth eruption and odontogenesis. The chemotherapeutic agents received between 1 and 5 years of age have negative impact on the rapidly dividing ameloblasts and odontoblasts, and the disorder of the ameloblast's production, the reduction of secretory function, the permeability of membrane and this can lead to the changes in calcium homeostasis. It causes inhibition of the formation of dentin, colchicine, vinblastine, which is dose dependent, of course. This was proved with animal experiments by Mataki et al. Moe et al. wrote three articles about the impact of vinblastine on ameloblasts in 1977 [93–96]. Lyaruu et al. studied the effect of actinomycin-D on the tooth development of hamsters, where it was found that depending on the size of the dose, the preodontoblasts necrotize, and the proliferation and differentiation do not occur. During their human studies, Hsieh et al. confirmed the results of Kaste et al., and noticed that above 7500 mg/m^2 of cyclophosphamide entry, there will be serious dental abnormalities [85, 97].

HSCT

Chronic GVHD occurs later in the transplant course, typically after day 100. Xerostomia, oral mucositis, and mucosal ulceration are frequent manifestations of chronic GVHD [98]. Dysphagia and pain on swallowing are common effects after HSCT [99–101]. Intensive chemotherapy and high-dose total body irradiation preceding SCT and young age at transplantation (that is mean before 6 years of age) lead to the worst dental and craniofacial late effects **Table 2.**

Calcification of permanent teeth begins after birth, taking 15–17 years (excluded third molars). After dental crown development, the cells of Hertwig epithelial root sheath initiate dental root development that can be seen on orthopantomogram or CBCT starting at age 3 years to 8 years. It is a slow and long process. The first sign of dental disturbances can be expected in 1–2 years. The same treatment can lead to dental agenesis or microdontia in an early age of life or tapered and blunted root later. The disturbing effect of HSCT is dependent on chemotherapeutic agents and irradiation. It has been revealed in animal and in vitro studies [96, 102, 103].

Decreased salivary function is a common finding in patients with GVHD who respond well to pilocarpine administration [39].

3.1. Impact of cancer therapy on tooth development

3.1.1. Delayed odontogenesis

Odontoblasts' activity decreases, which results in a change in the secretion of the microtubules, and thus resulting in a different tooth crowns` and roots` development.

The cronology of human dentition may vary between wide limits nevertheless among the cytostatic treatments' late side effect in delayed eruption and retention can be commonly seen.

Several controversial literatures can be found about the standard of the development of the teeth. One the most common and widest range was published by Kronfeld, in 1935, who dealt with the development of the teeth calcification. Kronfeld's modified chronology is used most widely.

During the development of enamel, because of the inducing effects of the predentin selected by the odontoblasts, the ameloblasts emits dentinenamel junction, which separates the enamel crystals and the dentin.

The ameloblasts' apical end is stretched and the granular texture of Tomes' processes is formed. This, peeled from the cell, gives the organic matrix of the enamel prism. This is followed by the calcification process, where millions of crystals deposit in the matrix—here hypomineralized enamel is formed due to the effect of cytostatics on the Ca balance) [104].

3.1.2. Dental disturbances

3.1.2.1. Enamel anomalies and hypoplasia

The cytostatic agents alter the cell cycle, the regeneration of ameloblast's reproduction, and the membrane's permeability. As a result of this process, an irregular surface of the enamel and enamel matrix is created, which changes the opacity of the enamel, and can lead to color differences and hypoplasia.

In the 80% of children who sustained remission but had been treated with chemotherapy, structural abnormalities was found in the enamel [105–107]. Vincristine, cyclophosphamide, and actinomycin can disturb the odontogenesis as well. Besides this, the amelogenesis also becomes impaired, which may create the emergence of hypomineralized enamel [96, 108, 109].

According a study by Alpaslan et al., among children treated with chemotherapy, the enamel discoloration's frequency was 57%, while in the healthy control group received no cancer treatment the enamel disturbance was 13%. Hypoplasia was observed among the 47% of the recovered children—this value was 15% among the healthy ones [110].

Oguz's study carried out in 2004 showed similar results. According to their study, the most common disorder was the enamel discoloration (67% vs. 25%) and enamel hypoplasia (56% vs. 44%) [111]. If the children were 5 years old or more at the time of the diagnosis of malignant tumors, the enamel discoloration (71%) and the hypoplasia (58%) were significantly higher [111].

Minicucci et al. showed the effect of cytostatic agents causing enamel anomalies. Among the 71 % of children treated with chemotherapy, detectable difference could be seen [112].

3.1.2.2. Dentin anomalies

Ayanoglou et al. examined the effect of cyclosporine A (CsA) in rats' molars. The reduction in dentin matrix mineralization and time prolongation was observed in the process, and as a consequence of this, lesions similar to dentinogenesis imperfecta starts in the dentin [57, 113].

The tooth development begins to form between the 6th and the 8th week of the prenatal development, and permanent tooth start to form in the 20th week and **can last until the 21th year** [114]. Thus, not only the in prenatal, but the postnatal diseases also can create serious malformations. The 4 years prior to the period of the tooth change are the most important and also the most critical period regarding the development of the permanent teeth. Chemotherapy given during this period has a negative impact on the rapidly dividing ameloblasts and odontoblasts. It can lead to malformations in the ameloblast's productions, decrease in the secretory functions, and changes in membrane permeability and the calcium homeostasis. Colchicine and vinblastine can cause inhibit the formation of dentine, which is dose dependent [93]. Moe et al. wrote three articles about the effect of vinblastine on ameloblasts in 1977 [95, 115]. Lyaruu et al. studied the effect of actinomycin-D on the tooth development of hamsters. They found that, depending on the size of the dose, the preodontoblasts necrotize. The proliferation and differentiation does not occur. Hsieh et al. confirmed the results of Kaste during their human studies saying that above 7500mg/m2 cyclophosphamide entry, there will be serious dental abnormalities [97].

Fromm et al. studied ear, nose and throat, ophthalmological, and dental differences of children with soft tissue sarcomas 5, 5 years after the completion of the treatment [79]. In 93% of the children, some dental abnormalities were found, and in 73%, there were short roots and agenesis. The decrease in parotid saliva production was detected in 23% of the cases.

In the study, the patients were not differentiated according to the treatment, so it is likely that the big difference was because of the children who underwent radiotherapy.

Estilo et al. investigated children diagnosed with head and neck region rhabdomyosarcoma [105]. Dental malformations were found in the case of 8 children from 10.

3.1.3. Anodontia and hypodontia

The hypodontia usually shows familiarity disorder. Acquired forms occur in children treated with radiation therapy or chemotherapy as the developing teeth are extremely sensitive to these chemical and physical disturbances.

Among children treated with chemotherapy, the frequency of hypodontia is supported by several international studies.

Alpaslan et al. found hypodontia among the 50% of children treated cytotoxic due to Hodgkin and non-Hodgkin's lymphoma [110]. Based on studies of Oguz et al., in which 36 children previously treated with chemotherapy for non-Hodgkin's lymphoma were observed, they found agenesis in the 44% of the test group, while in the control group, they found it in only 9 people that is 25% [111].

Kaste et al. found hypodontia in the half of 22 patients of rhabdomyosarcoma, and in 77% of the cases, other oral lesions were observed [84]. Kaste et al. observed 52 active children with neuroblastoma in the stage of tooth development. In 71% of them, dental deviations were detected and in 21%, hypodontia were observed [85].

Avsar et al. studied 96 malignant disease's survivor: agenesis was found in 19.8% [116]. Holtta et al. observed hypodontia of 31% between the 1-year survivors of benign and malignant tumors [117].

3.1.4. Microdontia

Microdontia is morphological anomalies the disorders in the size and shape of the teeth. In order to determine the tooth size differences, we compare these differences to the permanent teeth during the clinical tests. Garn et al. conducted a number of studies and determined the size of the average values of teeth in the second half of the last century [118, 119]. There are several tables about these figures in Wheeler's dental anatomy book.

One of the most common disorders in the size and shape of the teeth are the microdontia and taurodontismus (Appendix 1). These changes cause aesthetic, functional, and occlusion problems to the patient who needs professional dental care in adult's age.

The microdontia—similar to the hypodontia—is considered as a late side effect of radiation therapy, although several studies have shown that not only the X-ray radiation, but some cytostatics may cause microdontia, hypodontia, enamel hypoplasia, and root developmental differences (Appendix 1).

Minicucci et al. reported 76 children treated for cytotoxic drugs because of ALL [112]. From these data, it is clear that in childhood the cytostatic treatment received under the age of 6 years can cause microdontia.

Oguz et al. found microdontia in only 1 child from 36 children treated with chemotherapy due to NHL [111].

Jaffe et al. tested 68 patients who had been treated against cancer earlier. Twenty-three of them received only chemotherapy [77]. Based on their observations, higher incidence of the praemolaris' microdontia occurred in the group, which received cytostatic treatment earlier. This article does not mention the exact time, but most of the treatments could happen in the development of the premolars.

Nunn et al. [2, 120] during their examination found microdontia or indications in 27% cases of 52 children with hematology cancer. Less than a quarter of those children diagnosed with the malignant hematological disease received radiation, and this did not affect the head and neck region.

Höltta et al. observed the dental differences of children treated with neuroblastoma in their follow-up studies. Agenesis was observed in all members of the TBI group, while relevant differences occurred in 40% of the chemotherapy group [121]. Microdontia was found in 80% cases of children participating in the study [121].

3.1.5. Root malformation

3.1.5.1. Taurodontism

Taurodens is defined as a disorder when the molar tooth crown will extend at the expense of the roots, so the bifurcation (or trifurcation) is close to the root tips. This means that the tooth will be a column, which is based on divergent short. Cytostatics received in the early years of life prevent or slow the formation of Hertwig epithelial root sheath, thereby forming taurodens [122].

Kaste et al. examined 423 children treated with ALL cytotoxic drugs. In the case of 6 % of the children, taurodontism was observed [86].

Jaffe et al. also observed taurodontism in children after chemotherapy. They tested 23 children who received cytostatic treatment only, and they also showed microdontia and amelogenesis imperfecta differences [77].

Nunn et al. found taurodontism among the 27% of children treated with chemotherapy [120].

Lopes et al. found this lesion in 14% of the cases during the examination of 137 children with solid tumors and lymphoproliferative [123] (Appendix 1).

3.1.5.2. Thin, short, and tapered roots

The cytostatic agents change the ameloblast's reproduction which reduces the secretory function, the membrane permeability, and change calcium homeostasis. This could lead to disorders of enamel formation, which can result in the development of thin, short, and fragile roots. At the time of the tooth crown mineralization development, the root development begins. The crowns of the large incisors and the first molars can be seen on X-rays around at the age of three. As the tooth development is a long-term process, the lesions can be detected only after some years (Appendix 1).

The effects of cytostatic agents on the crown and root development have been supported with animal studies as well. Nasman et al. gave 13–30 mg/kg cyclophosphamide 1 ml of 0.9% NaCl to 18 between 3 and 10 days of age [124]. Disorders were found in the first and second molaris, and the third molars (wisdom) teeth of the rats in the SEM examinations. The first and second molar roots were shorter and thinner than the average. In the case of the third molars, there were not only differences in root development, but crown deficit was detected as well [125].

Rosenberg et al.'s investigation confirms that the root brevity and slow mineralization are frequent among children with cytostatic treatment frequent [126].

Oguz et al. found root deformation in 23 teeth of nine children from the examination of 36 children. Most of the anomalies were noticed in the lower central and lateral incisors, but the premolar and molar roots also showed lesion [111].

Alpaslan et al. observed premature apexification in the 6% of the patients, while other malformation affecting the roots occurred with 44% incidence [110]. Kaste et al. described that in 54% of 22 children treated with cytotoxic drugs due to rhabdomyosarcoma, some tooth root malformations were detected [86].

Marec-Berard et al. tested the dental developmental differences of children with Wilms' tumor depending on the duration of chemotherapy [127]. At least one tooth developmental difference was found in 70% of the examined children. Before this, in 2002, they tested children with Ewing sarcoma where in 50% of them, root malformations were found [128].

Rosenberg`s study examined 17 patients who received cytostatic agents because of ALL: in the case of 5 patients, the praemolaris' shortened roots were well demonstrated by X-ray, and in the case of 13 children, much thinner roots were found [126].

Runge et al. drew attention to the orthodontic difficulties due to the malformations in the root development. The high forces applied to the fixed devices can trigger external resorption in the above shorter roots [129].

3.2. Craniofacial effects

3.2.1. Osteoporosis and catch up growing

It was assumed that the chemotherapeutic agents affect the craniofacial development. The only question is that these consequences are temporary or permanent changes. Vincristine and doxorubicin experiments in young rats by Karsila et al. showed that the first vincristine injection has a crucial role in the skull development, but 100 days after the exposure, the lag is caught up [130]. The female rats regenerated significantly faster and achieved the development of the young rats not treated with chemotherapy. It was also found that all vincristine received rats' cranial values differ from the healthy control animals and the animals treated with doxorubicin. The length and height of the mandible, the front and rear face height is significantly different in the case of the vincristine-treated rats.

The serum levels of Ca and P is normal or low, after the chemotherapy treatment since the suppurative treatments include vitamin D and calcium supplementation. During 1–2 years of chemotherapy, the bones' mineral content is reduced so routine ultrasound bone measurements are done. After the treatment, an increased 'importing' growth starts; the growth curve is higher than the normal increment, so the vitamin D and calcium supplementation is important. The permanent tooth's development will be completed, however, and therefore shorter roots are established. After the end of the treatment, the bone age will be 1–1.5 years less compared to the chronological age, and the dental age will be 1–1.5 more years older.

http://dx.doi.org/10.5772/67040

Halton et al. found abnormal extremely low-1, 25 dihydroxyvitamin D3 synthesis with calciuria of ALL children, which caused the deficiency of calcium and phosphorus that reduced bone mineralization. The children undergone cancer treatment, especially if the protocol contained antifolate (MTX), alkylating agents (ifosfamide) or plain agents (cisplatin) [131, 132].

Fanconi syndrome (proximal tubular toxicity) can occur with calciuria and hypophosphatemia. ALL Halton and his co-s examined children treated with ALL, and found changes in bone mineralization, in the process of vitamin D metabolism and several skeletal discrepancies [132]. The amount of bone decrease and the risk of fractures increase. The bone hemostasis degrades because of the decrease in the resorption of the intestinal calcium and the increased calcium usage. Nesbit et al. wrote about this in 1976 [133]. They diagnosed the signs of osteoporosis. Clinicians try to maintain a balance with bisphosphonates, inhibiting the increased osteoclast activity that leads to osteolysis. They prevent the formation of macrophages, from monocytes; reduce the phagocytosis and cytokine production.

The bone growth of children with cancer and leukemia treatment is affected by the high dose and intensive steroid. It is very important to notice the damage on time. (e.g., fractures, cartilage formation disorder, and deformity). Certain chemotherapy treatments can affect hormone production, which leads to osteoporosis, or thinning bones (trabecular structure is maintained, but the quality varies). Although the hormone levels return to normal after treatment, the bone density does not return to normal level. Suitable calcium and vitamin D supplementation is necessary. Both osteoporosis and periodontitis are risk factors but these lesions were not reported in children. However, differences were found in the skull's development. Kaste's Working Group dealt with the issue of bone age, chronological age, and dental age. They found that the chronological age of the bone is lower and the dental age was significantly higher in children who underwent cancer therapy [134].

Karsila-Tenovuo et al. tested 40 children; in the 1st group, there were 18 children who received 1 cranial irradiation and chemotherapy, eight of them got hormone therapy. In the 2nd group, there were 11 children with extracranial solid tumor treated with alkylating agents, while 11 children with Wilms' tumor belonged to Group 3 who received only chemotherapy [135].

Normal growth was found in the second group. In the group 3, the cephalometria results remained within the normal range, except for certain details of the maxilla and the rear face height [135].

4. Common Toxicity Criteria

The WHO Common Toxicity Criteria (CTC) was founded in 1999; it currently has 4:03 version in force, which was modified in 2010 under the name Common Terminology Criteria for Adverse Events (CTCAE). The table is included in the "Gastrointestinal System Differences" cheilitis and gingivitis, lip pain, mucositis, oral fistula, pain, periodontal disease, dental mal formations, dental pain, "Systemic side effects", the facial pain, "Infectious Diseases" the gingivitis, the lips, mucous and infectious diseases, sinusitis salivary glands. In the "musculoskeletal system diseases," the mouth bone necrosis and trismus, in the "The neurological lesions" the dysgeusia, the mimical- and chewing muscle weakness, facial nerve lesions, trigeminal neuralgia, and sinus pain, and in the "Skin and subcutaneous lesions," the oral cavity, erythema multiforme, pruritus, and purpura were included.

5. Follow-up guidelines for survivors of childhood, adolescent, and young adult cancers

All children undergoing high-dose chemotherapy and/or radiotherapy or SCT should be referred for dental and oral hygiene assessment prior to commencement of therapy. All children with diagnosis of malignant disease should be encouraged to maintain good oral hygiene, which requires not only tooth brushing but proper oral hygiene during and after anticancer therapy. Our guidelines are shown in **Figure 1**.

It is important to know the possible side effects encountered in the treatment. The family must be provided with the proper advice according to the changed life situation (daily routine, nutrition, oral and dental hygiene). The play specialist has an important role in facilitating the child`s understanding of cancer therapy. They make use of various types of play and game depending on the child's needs, age, culture issues, and understanding to provide information about hospitalization and teach new information [136, 137].

During the treatment, a specialized team (dental hygienist) should monitor the daily oral hygiene routine for children, as many banal and painful infections can be prevented.

The oral hygiene habits should be immediately restored after the completion of therapy, in order not to increase the serious side effects.

In my opinion, the children undergone cancer therapy should be controlled in every 3 months during the first year, but from the next year, it does not have to be more frequent, rather more thorough and accurately documented. The most important is that parents do not have to forget the necessary check-ups.

The dental care of children with malignant disease does not differ from the healthy ones, except for the invasive interventions. It would be interesting and obvious that children cancer patients should belong to territorial care pedodontists, but unfortunately the current children's dental network is not suitable in many countries for this because the children will not receive effective care.

It would be worth to follow and treat them in the university center, near the oncology centers. It will be good to create a patient card, where the dental status of the survivors could be followed.

It is important to mention here that cooperation between pediatric clinics and dental clinics should be encouraged to enforce the implication of oral preventive measures for children in chemotherapy in a way to improve their oral health. Clinicians and dentist should provide treatment to improve both the oral hygiene and the nutritional status of children cancer survivors.

http://dx.doi.org/10.5772/67040

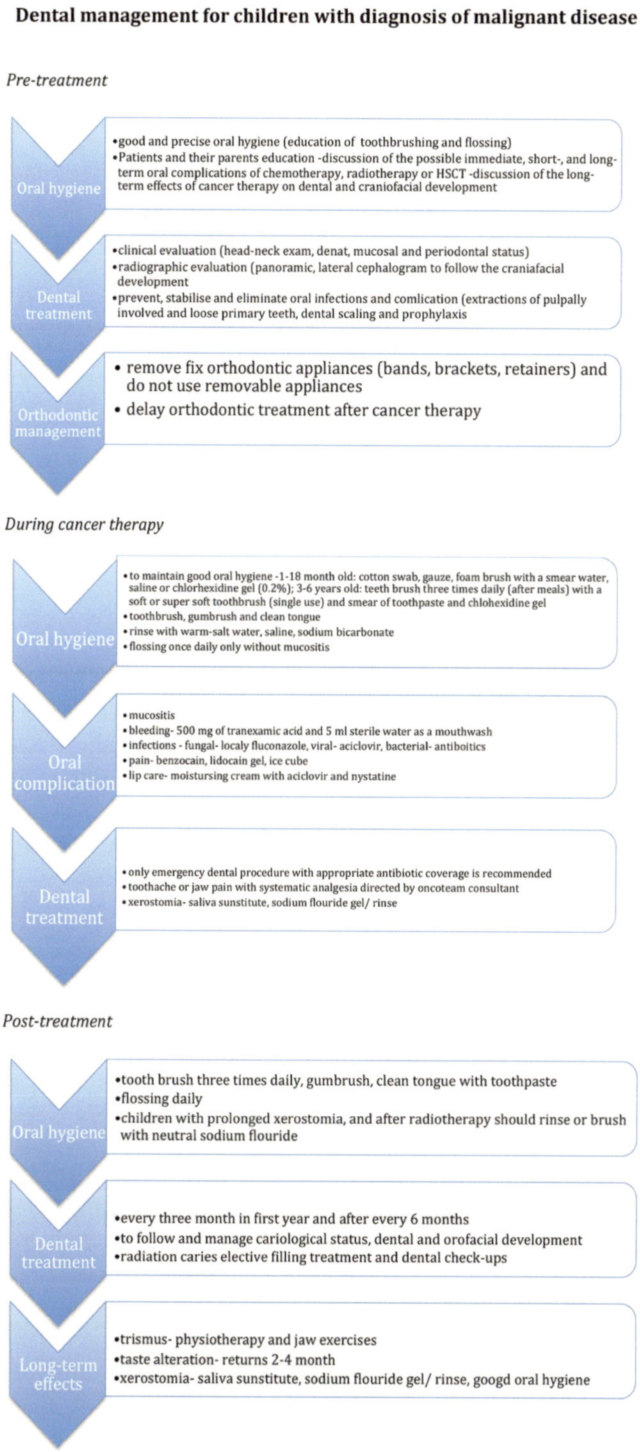

Figure 1. Dental management for children with diagnosis of malignant disease.

Appendix 1

Disturbances

Delayed odontogenesis

The cronology of human dentition may vary between wide limits nevertheless among the cytostatic treatments' late side effect in dentitio tarda and retention dentis can be commonly seen.

The most sensitive age for dental disturbances is 2–5 years of age. Microdontia (orange arrows), Delayed eruption of second premolar (blue arrow).

Shape and size of teeth

The most frequented anomalies of shape and size of teeth development are microdontia (blue circles) and aplasia.

Disturbances

Microdontia

Microdontia is in the most of cases late effects of radiotherapy.

Thin, short, and tapered roots

Late effects of cancer therapy are anomalies of root development (blue circles).

Taurodens

Taurodens is defined as a disorder when the molar tooth crown will extend at the expense of the roots, so (red circles).

Disturbances

Delayed eruption of second premolars.
Taurodens of first molars.

Abbreviation

5-FU	Fluorouracil, a drug used in medicine
ALL	Acute lymphoblastic leukemia
Ca	Calcium
CBCT	Cone beam computed tomography
CTCAE	Common Terminology Criteria for Adverse Events
CsA	Cyclosporin A
DEJ	Dentinoenamel junction

DMF-T index	Decay-missing-filled index, a quantification of dental caries burden
GVHD	Graft-versus-host disease
Gy	Gray, SI unit of absorbed radiation
HNC	Head and neck cancer
HSCT	Hematopoietic stem cell transplantation
MTX	Methotrexate, a drug used in medicine
NHL	Non-Hodgkin lymphoma
P	Phosphorus
pH	Numeric scale used to specify the acidity or basicity of an aqueous solution
RT	Radiation therapy
SCT	Stem cell transplantation
TBI	A form of radiation therapy used most commonly in bone marrow transplantation
WHO CTC	World Health Organization Common Toxicity Criteria

Author details

Orsolya Németh

Address all correspondence to: drnemethorsolya@gmail.com

Department of Community Dentistry, Semmelweis University, Budapest, Hungary

References

[1] Melsen B. Palatal growth studied on human autopsy material. A histologic microradiographic study. Am J Orthod. 1975;68(1):42–54.

[2] Persson M, Thilander B. Palatal suture closure in man from 15 to 35 years of age. Am J Orthod. 1977;72(1):42–52.

[3] Enlow DH, BANG S. Growth and remodeling of the human maxilla. Am J Orthod. 1965;51:446–64.

[4] Carlson DS, Buschang P. Craniofacial growth and development: evidence-based perspectives. In: Graber LW, Vanarsdall RL, Vig KWL, editors. Orthodontics Current Principles and Techniques. Philadelphia: Elsevier Mosby; 2012. pp. 215–43.

[5] Sarnat BG, Shanedling PD. Postnatal growth of the orbit and upper face in rabbits after exenteration of the orbit. Arch Ophthalmol. 1965;73:829–37.

[6] Ten Cate AR. Development of the tooth and its supporting tissues. In: Ten Cate AR, editor. Oral Histology Development, Structure and Function. Missuri: Mosby; 1985. pp. 56–77.

[7] Petrovic AG, Oudet CL, Shaye R. [Mandible positioning with a maxillary activator appliance with lateral occlusal blocks of various heights in relation to daily treatment time]. Fortschr Kieferorthop. 1982;43(4):243–70.

[8] Lavergne J, Petrovic A. Discontinuities in occlusal relationship and the regulation of facial growth. A cybernetic view. Eur J Orthod. 1983;5(4):269–78.

[9] McNamara JA, Carlson DS. Quantitative analysis of temporomandibular joint adaptations to protrusive function. Am J Orthod. 1979;76(6):593–611.

[10] Sandler TW. Head and Neck. In: Sandler TW, editor. Langman`s Medical Embriology. Philadelphia: Lippincott Wiliams & Wilkins; 2012. pp. 260–87.

[11] Ten Cate AR. Dentinogenesis. In: Ten Cate AR, editor. Oral Histology Development, Stucture and Function. Missouri: Mosby; 1985. pp. 129–46.

[12] Kun L, Moulder J. General principles of radiation therapy. In: Poplack DG, Pizzo AP, editors. Principles and Practice of Pediatric Oncology. Philadelphia: J.B. Lippincott Company; 1993. pp. 273–303.

[13] Doline S, Needleman HL, Petersen RA, Cassady JR. The effect of radiotherapy in the treatment of retinoblastoma upon the developing dentition. J Pediatr Ophthalmol Strabismus. 1980;17(2):109–13.

[14] Rubin P. The Franz Buschke lecture: late effects of chemotherapy and radiation therapy: a new hypothesis. Int J Radiat Oncol Biol Phys. 1984;10(1):5–34.

[15] Naidu MU, Ramana GV, Rani PU, Mohan IK, Suman A, Roy P. Chemotherapy-induced and/or radiation therapy-induced oral mucositis--complicating the treatment of cancer. Neoplasia. 2004;6(5):423–31.

[16] Epstein JB, Loh R, Stevenson-Moore P, McBride BC, Spinelli J. Chlorhexidine rinse in prevention of dental caries in patients following radiation therapy. Oral Surg Oral Med Oral Pathol. 1989;68(4):401–5.

[17] Keene HJ, Daly T, Brown LR, Dreizen S, Drane JB, Horton IM, et al. Dental caries and *Streptococcus mutans* prevalence in cancer patients with irradiation-induced xerostomia: 1–13 years after radiotherapy. Caries Res. 1981;15(5):416–27.

[18] Kielbassa AM, Hellwig E, Meyer-Lueckel H. Effects of irradiation on in situ remineralization of human and bovine enamel demineralized in vitro. Caries Res. 2006;40(2):130–5.

[19] Kielbassa AM, Hinkelbein W, Hellwig E, Meyer-Lückel H. Radiation-related damage to dentition. Lancet Oncol. 2006;7(4):326–35.

[20] Epstein JB, Chin EA, Jacobson JJ, Rishiraj B, Le N. The relationships among fluoride, cariogenic oral flora, and salivary flow rate during radiation therapy. Oral Surg Oral Med Oral Pathol Oral Radiol Endod. 1998;86(3):286–92.

[21] Springer IN, Niehoff P, Warnke PH, Böcek G, Kovács G, Suhr M, et al. Radiation caries–radiogenic destruction of dental collagen. Oral Oncol. 2005;41(7):723–8.

[22] Spiegel RJ. The acute toxicities of chemotherapy. Cancer Treat Rev. 1981;8(3):197–207.

[23] Blatt J, Bleyer A, D C. Late effects of childhood cancer and its treatment. In: Pizzo, Philip A., and David G. Poplack editors. Principles and Practice of Pediatric Oncology. 6th ed. Philadelphia: J. B. Lippincott Company; 1993. p. 1091–114.

[24] Wong KY, Lampkin BC. Anthracycline toxicity. Am J Pediatr Hematol Oncol. 1983;5(1):93–7.

[25] Eghbali A, Taherkhanchi B, Bagheri B, Sadeghi Sedeh B. Effect of chewing gum on oral mucositis in children undergoing chemotherapy: a randomized controlled study. Iran J Ped Hematol Oncol. 2016;6(1):9–14.

[26] Pixberg C, Koch R, Eich HT, Martinsson U, Kristensen I, Matuschek C, et al. Acute toxicity grade 3 and 4 after irradiation in children and adolescents: results from the IPPARCA collaboration. Int J Radiat Oncol Biol Phys. 2016;94(4):792–9.

[27] Bardellini E, Amadori F, Majorana A. Oral hygiene grade and quality of life in children with chemotherapy-related oral mucositis: a randomized study on the impact of a fluoride toothpaste with salivary enzymes, essential oils, proteins and colostrum extract versus a fluoride toothpaste without menthol. Int J Dent Hyg. 2016.

[28] Bardellini E, Amadori F, Schumacher RF, D'Ippolito C, Porta F, Majorana A. Efficacy of a solution composed by verbascoside, polyvinylpyrrolidone (PVP) and sodium hyaluronate in the treatment of chemotherapy-induced oral mucositis in children with acute lymphoblastic leukemia. J Pediatr Hematol Oncol. 2016.

[29] Bardellini E, Schumacher F, Conti G, Porta F, Campus G, Majorana A. Risk factors for oral mucositis in children receiving hematopoietic cell transplantation for primary immunodeficiencies: a retrospective study. Pediatr Transplant. 2013;17(5):492–7.

[30] Bleyer WA. The clinical pharmacology of methotrexate: new applications of an old drug. Cancer. 1978;41(1):36–51.

[31] Sonis AL. Craniofacial development, teeth and salivary glands. In: Daniel Green, Hamish Wallace, editors. Late effects of childhood cancer. 1st ed. London: Arnold; 2004. p. 176–86.

[32] Gupta A, West HJ. Mucositis (or Stomatitis). JAMA Oncol. 2016.

[33] Ribeiro RA, Wanderley CW, Wong DV, Mota JM, Leite CA, Souza MH, et al. Irinotecan- and 5-fluorouracil-induced intestinal mucositis: insights into pathogenesis and therapeutic perspectives. Cancer Chemother Pharmacol. 2016.

[34] Keefe DM, Rassias G, O'Neil L, Gibson RJ. Severe mucositis: how can nutrition help? Curr Opin Clin Nutr Metab Care. 2007;10(5):627–31.

[35] Riley P, McCabe MG, Glenny AM. Oral cryotherapy for preventing oral mucositis in patients receiving cancer treatment. JAMA Oncol. 2016.

[36] Sonesson M. On minor salivary gland secretion in children, adolescents and adults. Swed Dent J Suppl. 2011(215):9–64.

[37] Sonesson M, Eliasson L, Matsson L. Minor salivary gland secretion in children and adults. Arch Oral Biol. 2003;48(7):535–9.

[38] Köstler WJ, Hejna M, Wenzel C, Zielinski CC. Oral mucositis complicating chemotherapy and/or radiotherapy: options for prevention and treatment. CA Cancer J Clin. 2001;51(5):290–315.

[39] Fox PC, van der Ven PF, Baum BJ, Mandel ID. Pilocarpine for the treatment of xerostomia associated with salivary gland dysfunction. Oral Surg Oral Med Oral Pathol. 1986;61(3):243–8.

[40] Belfield PM, Dwyer AA. Oral complications of childhood cancer and its treatment: current best practice. Eur J Cancer. 2004;40(7):1035–41; discussion 42–4.

[41] Nemeth O, Kivovics M, Pinke I, Marton K, Kivovics P, Garami M. Late effects of multiagent chemotherapy on salivary secretion in children cancer survivors. J Am Coll Nutr. 2014;33(3):186–91.

[42] Lee SK, Lee SW, Chung SC, Kim YK, Kho HS. Analysis of residual saliva and minor salivary gland secretions in patients with dry mouth. Arch Oral Biol. 2002;47(9):637–41.

[43] Lee YL, Santacroce SJ. Posttraumatic stress in long-term young adult survivors of childhood cancer: a questionnaire survey. Int J Nurs Stud. 2007;44(8):1406–17.

[44] Ribelles Llop M, Guinot Jimeno F, Mayné Acién R, Bellet Dalmau LJ. Effects of xylitol chewing gum on salivary flow rate, pH, buffering capacity and presence of Streptococcus mutans in saliva. Eur J Paediatr Dent. 2010;11(1):9–14.

[45] Barbería E, Hernandez C, Miralles V, Maroto M. Paediatric patients receiving oncology therapy: review of the literature and oral management guidelines. Eur J Paediatr Dent. 2008;9(4):188–94.

[46] Committee AAoPDCA, Affairs AAoPDCoC. Guideline on dental management of pediatric patients receving chemotherapy, hematopoietic cell transplantation, and/or radiation. Pediatr Dent. 2008;30(7 Suppl):219–25.

[47] Sheller B, Williams B. Orthodontic management of patients with hematologic malignancies. Am J Orthod Dentofacial Orthop. 1996;109(6):575–80.

[48] Singh N, Scully C, Joyston-Bechal S. Oral complications of cancer therapies: prevention and management. Clin Oncol (R Coll Radiol). 1996;8(1):15–24.

[49] Welbury RR, Craft AW, Murray JJ, Kernahan J. Dental health of survivors of malignant disease. Arch Dis Child. 1984;59(12):1186–7.

[50] Alberth M, Kovalecz G, Nemes J, Máth J, Kiss C, Márton IJ. Oral health of long-term childhood cancer survivors. Pediatr Blood Cancer. 2004;43(1):88–90.

[51] Alberth M, Majoros L, Kovalecz G, Borbás E, Szegedi I, J Márton I, et al. Significance of oral candida infections in children with cancer. Pathol Oncol Res. 2006;12(4):237–41.

[52] Dens F, Boute P, Otten J, Vinckier F, Declerck D. Dental caries, gingival health, and oral hygiene of long term survivors of paediatric malignant diseases. Arch Dis Child. 1995;72(2):129–32.

[53] Dens FL, Boute P, Vinckier F, Declerck D. Salivary caries risk factors in long-term event-free survivors of pediatric malignant diseases. J Clin Pediatr Dent. 1996;20(3):241–5.

[54] Pajari U, Larmas M, Lanning M. Caries incidence and prevalence in children receiving antineoplastic therapy. Caries Res. 1988;22(5):318–20.

[55] Pajari U, Ollila P, Lanning M. Incidence of dental caries in children with acute lymphoblastic leukemia is related to the therapy used. ASDC J Dent Child. 1995;62(5):349–52.

[56] Sonis AL, Waber DP, Sallan S, Tarbell NJ. The oral health of long-term survivors of acute lymphoblastic leukaemia: a comparison of three treatment modalities. Eur J Cancer B Oral Oncol. 1995;31B(4):250–2.

[57] Ayanoglou CM, Godeau G, Lesty C, Septier D, Goldberg M. Cyclosporin A-induced alterations of dentinogenesis in rat molars. J Oral Pathol Med. 1997;26(3):129–34.

[58] Squier CA. Oral complications of cancer therapies. Mucosal alterations. NCI Monogr. 1990(9):169–72.

[59] Askins MA, Moore BD. Preventing neurocognitive late effects in childhood cancer survivors. J Child Neurol. 2008;23(10):1160–71.

[60] Askins MA, Moore BD. Psychosocial support of the pediatric cancer patient: lessons learned over the past 50 years. Curr Oncol Rep. 2008;10(6):469–76.

[61] Bielack SS, Rerin JS, Dickerhoff R, Dilloo D, Kremens B, von Stackelberg A, et al. Osteosarcoma after allogeneic bone marrow transplantation. A report of four cases from the Cooperative Osteosarcoma Study Group (COSS). Bone Marrow Transplant. 2003; 31(5):353–9.

[62] Challinor J, Miaskowski C, Moore I, Slaughter R, Franck L. Review of research studies that evaluated the impact of treatment for childhood cancers on neurocognition and behavioral and social competence: nursing implications. J Soc Pediatr Nurs. 2000;5(2):57–74.

[63] de Moor JS, Mariotto AB, Parry C, Alfano CM, Padgett L, Kent EE, et al. Cancer survivors in the United States: prevalence across the survivorship trajectory and implications for care. Cancer Epidemiol Biomarkers Prev. 2013;22(4):561–70.

[64] De Moor R. [Direct and indirect effects of medication (including chemotherapy) and irradiation on the pulp]. Rev Belge Med Dent (1984). 2000;55(4):321–33.

[65] Hockenberry M, Krull K, Moore K, Gregurich MA, Casey ME, Kaemingk K. Longitudinal evaluation of fine motor skills in children with leukemia. J Pediatr Hematol Oncol. 2007;29(8):535–9.

[66] Kaemingk KL, Carey ME, Moore IM, Herzer M, Hutter JJ. Math weaknesses in survivors of acute lymphoblastic leukemia compared to healthy children. Child Neuropsychol. 2004;10(1):14–23.

[67] Ki Moore IM, Hockenberry MJ, Krull KR. Cancer-related cognitive changes in children, adolescents and adult survivors of childhood cancers. Semin Oncol Nurs. 2013;29(4):248–59.

[68] Krull KR, Hockenberry MJ, Miketova P, Carey M, Moore IM. Chemotherapy-related changes in central nervous system phospholipids and neurocognitive function in childhood acute lymphoblastic leukemia. Leuk Lymphoma. 2013;54(3):535–40.

[69] Nathan PC, Patel SK, Dilley K, Goldsby R, Harvey J, Jacobsen C, et al. Guidelines for identification of, advocacy for, and intervention in neurocognitive problems in survivors of childhood cancer: a report from the Children's Oncology Group. Arch Pediatr Adolesc Med. 2007;161(8):798–806.

[70] Grundy RG, Wilne SH, Robinson KJ, Ironside JW, Cox T, Chong WK, et al. Primary postoperative chemotherapy without radiotherapy for treatment of brain tumours other than ependymoma in children under 3 years: results of the first UKCCSG/SIOP CNS 9204 trial. Eur J Cancer. 2010;46(1):120–33.

[71] Mitchell C, Pritchard-Jones K, Shannon R, Hutton C, Stevens S, Machin D, et al. Immediate nephrectomy versus preoperative chemotherapy in the management of non-metastatic Wilms' tumour: results of a randomised trial (UKW3) by the UK Children's Cancer Study Group. Eur J Cancer. 2006;42(15):2554–62.

[72] Reed R, Xu C, Liu Y, Gorski JP, Wang Y, Walker MP. Radiotherapy effect on nano-mechanical properties and chemical composition of enamel and dentine. Arch Oral Biol. 2015;60(5):690–7.

[73] Sanpakit K, Triwatanawong J, Sumboonnanonda A. Long-term outcome in pediatric renal tumor survivors: experience of a single center. J Pediatr Hematol Oncol. 2013;35(8):610–3.

[74] Walker DA. Health status measures in young people's cancer trials; a time to move health-related quality of life up to primary outcome measures. Qual Life Res. 2006;15(1):159–60.

[75] Walker MP, Wichman B, Cheng AL, Coster J, Williams KB. Impact of radiotherapy dose on dentition breakdown in head and neck cancer patients. Pract Radiat Oncol. 2011;1(3):142–8.

[76] Nishihori T, Shirato H, Aoyama H, Onimaru R, Komae T, Ishii N, et al. Three-dimensional conformal radiotherapy for astrocytic tumors involving the eloquent area in children and young adults. J Neurooncol. 2002;60(2):177–83.

[77] Jaffe N, Toth BB, Hoar RE, Ried HL, Sullivan MP, McNeese MD. Dental and maxillofacial abnormalities in long-term survivors of childhood cancer: effects of treatment with chemotherapy and radiation to the head and neck. Pediatrics. 1984;73(6):816–23.

[78] Kaste SC, Goodman P, Leisenring W, Stovall M, Hayashi RJ, Yeazel M, et al. Impact of radiation and chemotherapy on risk of dental abnormalities: a report from the Childhood Cancer Survivor Study. Cancer. 2009;115(24):5817–27.

[79] Fromm M, Littman P, Raney RB, Nelson L, Handler S, Diamond G, et al. Late effects after treatment of twenty children with soft tissue sarcomas of the head and neck. Experience at a single institution with a review of the literature. Cancer. 1986;57(10):2070–6.

[80] Cubukçu CE, Sevinir B. Dental health indices of long-term childhood cancer survivors who had oral supervision during treatment: a case-control study. Pediatr Hematol Oncol. 2008;25(7):638–46.

[81] Cubukcu CE, Sevinir B, Ercan I. Disturbed dental development of permanent teeth in children with solid tumors and lymphomas. Pediatr Blood Cancer. 2012;58(1):80–4.

[82] Hölttä P, Hovi L, Saarinen-Pihkala UM, Peltola J, Alaluusua S. Disturbed root development of permanent teeth after pediatric stem cell transplantation. Dental root development after SCT. Cancer. 2005;103(7):1484–93.

[83] Hong CH, Napeñas JJ, Hodgson BD, Stokman MA, Mathers-Stauffer V, Elting LS, et al. A systematic review of dental disease in patients undergoing cancer therapy. Support Care Cancer. 2010;18(8):1007–21.

[84] Kaste SC, Hopkins KP, Bowman LC. Dental abnormalities in long-term survivors of head and neck rhabdomyosarcoma. Med Pediatr Oncol. 1995;25(2):96–101.

[85] Kaste SC, Hopkins KP, Bowman LC, Santana VM. Dental abnormalities in children treated for neuroblastoma. Med Pediatr Oncol. 1998;30(1):22–7.

[86] Kaste SC, Hopkins KP, Jones D, Crom D, Greenwald CA, Santana VM. Dental abnormalities in children treated for acute lymphoblastic leukemia. Leukemia. 1997;11(6):792–6.

[87] Kawakami T, Nakamura Y, Karibe H. Cyclophosphamide-induced morphological changes in dental root development of ICR mice. PLoS One. 2015;10(7):e0133256.

[88] Stanisavljevic S, Babcock AL. Fractures in children treated with methotrexate for leukemia. Clin Orthop Relat Res. 1977(125):139–44.

[89] Ecklund K, Laor T, Goorin AM, Connolly LP, Jaramillo D. Methotrexate osteopathy in patients with osteosarcoma. Radiology. 1997;202(2):543–7.

[90] Pennes DR, Ellis CN, Madison KC, Voorhees JJ, Martel W. Early skeletal hyperostoses secondary to 13-cis-retinoic acid. AJR Am J Roentgenol. 1984;142(5):979–83.

[91] Reade PC, Roberts ML. Some long-term effects of cyclophosphamide on the growth of rat incisor teeth. Arch Oral Biol. 1978;23(11):1001–5.

[92] Burn-Murdoch RA. The effect of corticosteroids and cyclophosphamide on the eruption of resected incisor teeth in the rat. Arch Oral Biol. 1988;33(9):661–7.

[93] Mataki S. Comparison of the effect of colchicine and vinblastine on the inhibiton of dentinogenesis in rat incisors. Arch Oral Biol. 1981;26(12):955–61.

[94] Moe H, Mikkelsen H. On the effect of vinblastine on ameloblasts of rat incisors in vivo. 2. Protracted effect on secretory ameloblasts. A light microscopical study. Acta Pathol Microbiol Scand A. 1977;85(3):319–29.

[95] Moe H, Mikkelsen H. Light microscopical and ultrastructural observations on the effect of vinblastine on ameloblasts of rat incisors in vivo. I. Short-term effect on secretory ameloblasts. Acta Pathol Microbiol Scand A. 1977;85A(1):73–88.

[96] Lyaruu DM, van Duin MA, Bervoets TJ, Wöltgens JH, Bronckers AL. Effects of vincristine on the developing hamster tooth germ in vitro. Connect Tissue Res. 1995;32(1–4):281–9.

[97] Hsieh SG, Hibbert S, Shaw P, Ahern V, Arora M. Association of cyclophosphamide use with dental developmental defects and salivary gland dysfunction in recipients of childhood antineoplastic therapy. Cancer. 2011;117(10):2219–27.

[98] Schubert MM, Correa ME. Oral graft-versus-host disease. Dent Clin North Am. 2008;52(1):79–109, viii–ix.

[99] Rodu B, Gockerman JP. Oral manifestations of the chronic graft-v-host reaction. JAMA. 1983;249(4):504–7.

[100] Sullivan KM. Longterm followup and quality of life after hematopoietic stem cell transplantation. J Rheumatol Suppl. 1997;48:46–52.

[101] Barrett AJ, Le Blanc K. Prophylaxis of acute GVHD: manipulate the graft or the environment? Best Pract Res Clin Haematol. 2008;21(2):165–76.

[102] Stene T, Koppang HS. Autoradiographic investigation of proliferative responses in rat incisor pulp after vincristine administration. Scand J Dent Res. 1980;88(2):96–103.

[103] Dahllöf G. Oral and dental late effects after pediatric stem cell transplantation. Biol Blood Marrow Transplant. 2008;14(1 Suppl 1):81–3.

[104] Kaste SC, Hopkins KP, Jenkins JJ. Abnormal odontogenesis in children treated with radiation and chemotherapy: imaging findings. AJR Am J Roentgenol. 1994;162(6):1407–11.

[105] Estilo CL, Huryn JM, Kraus DH, Sklar CA, Wexler LH, Wolden SL, et al. Effects of therapy on dentofacial development in long-term survivors of head and neck rhabdomyosarcoma: the memorial sloan-kettering cancer center experience. J Pediatr Hematol Oncol. 2003;25(3):215–22.

[106] Maciel JC, de Castro CG, Brunetto AL, Di Leone LP, da Silveira HE. Oral health and dental anomalies in patients treated for leukemia in childhood and adolescence. Pediatr Blood Cancer. 2009;53(3):361–5.

[107] Purdell-Lewis DJ, Stalman MS, Leeuw JA, Humphrey GB, Kalsbeek H. Long term results of chemotherapy on the developing dentition: caries risk and developmental aspects. Community Dent Oral Epidemiol. 1988;16(2):68–71.

[108] Dahl JE. Immediate and delayed effects of repeated doxorubicin injections on rat incisor mesenchymal cells. Acta Odontol Scand. 1985;43(3):155–62.

[109] Vahlsing HL, Feringa ER, Britten AG, Kinning WK. Dental abnormalities in rats after a single large dose of cyclophosphamide. Cancer Res. 1975;35(8):2199–202.

[110] Alpaslan G, Alpaslan C, Gögen H, Oğuz A, Cetiner S, Karadeniz C. Disturbances in oral and dental structures in patients with pediatric lymphoma after chemotherapy: a preliminary report. Oral Surg Oral Med Oral Pathol Oral Radiol Endod. 1999;87(3):317–21.

[111] Oğuz A, Cetiner S, Karadeniz C, Alpaslan G, Alpaslan C, Pinarli G. Long-term effects of chemotherapy on orodental structures in children with non-Hodgkin's lymphoma. Eur J Oral Sci. 2004;112(1):8–11.

[112] Minicucci EM, Lopes LF, Crocci AJ. Dental abnormalities in children after chemotherapy treatment for acute lymphoid leukemia. Leuk Res. 2003;27(1):45–50.

[113] Ayanoglou CM, Lesty C. Maintenance of new cementum formed during cyclosporin A administration after suspension of the treatment. J Periodontal Res. 1997;32(7):614–8.

[114] Sadler TW. Langman's Medical Embryology. 12th ed. Philadelphia, Lippincott Williams & Wilkins a Wolters Kluver; 2012.

[115] Moe H. On the effect of vinblastine on ameloblasts of rat incisors in vivo. 3. Acute and protracted effect on differentiating ameloblasts. A light microscopical study. Acta Pathol Microbiol Scand A. 1977;85(3):330–4.

[116] Avşar A, Elli M, Darka O, Pinarli G. Long-term effects of chemotherapy on caries formation, dental development, and salivary factors in childhood cancer survivors. Oral Surg Oral Med Oral Pathol Oral Radiol Endod. 2007;104(6):781–9.

[117] Hölttä P, Alaluusua S, Saarinen-Pihkala UM, Peltola J, Hovi L. Agenesis and microdontia of permanent teeth as late adverse effects after stem cell transplantation in young children. Cancer. 2005;103(1):181–90.

[118] Garn SM, Lewis AB, Kerewsky RS. Size interrelationships of the mesial and distal teeth. J Dent Res. 1965;44:350–4.

[119] Garn SM, Lewis AB, Kerewsky RS. Genetic, nutritional, and maturational correlates of dental development. J Dent Res. 1965;44:Suppl:228–42.

[120] Nunn JH, Welbury RR, Gordon PH, Kernahan J, Craft AW. Dental caries and dental anomalies in children treated by chemotherapy for malignant disease: a study in the north of England. Int J Paediatr Dent. 1991;1(3):131–5.

[121] Hölttä P, Alaluusua S, Saarinen-Pihkala UM, Wolf J, Nyström M, Hovi L. Long-term adverse effects on dentition in children with poor-risk neuroblastoma treated with high-dose chemotherapy and autologous stem cell transplantation with or without total body irradiation. Bone Marrow Transplant. 2002;29(2):121–7.

[122] Goho C. Chemoradiation therapy: effect on dental development. Pediatr Dent. 1993;15(1):6–12.

[123] Lopes NN, Petrilli AS, Caran EM, França CM, Chilvarquer I, Lederman H. Dental abnormalities in children submitted to antineoplastic therapy. J Dent Child (Chic). 2006;73(3):140–5.

[124] Näsman M, Hammarström L. Influence of the antineoplastic agent cyclophosphamide on dental development in rat molars. Acta Odontol Scand. 1996;54(5):287–94.

[125] Näsman M, Forsberg CM, Dahllöf G. Long-term dental development in children after treatment for malignant disease. Eur J Orthod. 1997;19(2):151–9.

[126] Rosenberg SW, Kolodney H, Wong GY, Murphy ML. Altered dental root development in long-term survivors of pediatric acute lymphoblastic leukemia. A review of 17 cases. Cancer. 1987;59(9):1640–8.

[127] Marec-Berard P, Azzi D, Chaux-Bodard AG, Lagrange H, Gourmet R, Bergeron C. Long-term effects of chemotherapy on dental status in children treated for nephroblastoma. Pediatr Hematol Oncol. 2005;22(7):581–8.

[128] Marec-Berard P, Bergeron C, Frappaz D, Philip T, Gorry F, Chaux-Bodard AG, et al. [Anomalies of dental development in children receiving chemotherapy]. Arch Pediatr. 2002;9(11):1212–3.

[129] Runge ME, Edwards DL. Orthodontic treatment for an adolescent with a history of acute lymphoblastic leukemia. Pediatr Dent. 2000;22(6):494–8.

[130] Karsila S, Salmi T, Helenius H, Rönning O. Craniofacial growth of immature rats following administration of vincristine and doxorubicin. Eur J Orthod. 2000;22(5):545–53.

[131] Halton JM, Atkinson SA, Fraher L, Webber C, Gill GJ, Dawson S, et al. Altered mineral metabolism and bone mass in children during treatment for acute lymphoblastic leukemia. J Bone Miner Res. 1996;11(11):1774–83.

[132] Halton JM, Atkinson SA, Fraher L, Webber CE, Cockshott WP, Tam C, et al. Mineral homeostasis and bone mass at diagnosis in children with acute lymphoblastic leukemia. J Pediatr. 1995;126(4):557–64.

[133] Nesbit M, Krivit W, Heyn R, Sharp H. Acute and chronic effects of methotrexate on hepatic, pulmonary, and skeletal systems. Cancer. 1976;37(2 Suppl):1048–57.

[134] Kaste SC, Jones-Wallace D, Rose SR, Boyett JM, Lustig RH, Rivera GK, et al. Bone mineral decrements in survivors of childhood acute lymphoblastic leukemia: frequency of occurrence and risk factors for their development. Leukemia. 2001;15(5):728–34.

[135] Karsila-Tenovuo S, Jahnukainen K, Peltomäki T, Minn H, Kulmala J, Salmi TT, et al. Disturbances in craniofacial morphology in children treated for solid tumors. Oral Oncol. 2001;37(7):586–92.

[136] Vessey JA, Mahon MM. Therapeutic play and the hospitalized child. J Pediatr Nurs. 1990;5(5):328–33.

[137] Webster NR, Galley HF. Nutrition in the critically ill patient. J R Coll Surg Edinb. 2000;45(6):373–9.

Chapter 3

Used of Complementary and Alternative Medicine on Symptoms Management and Quality of Life

Ayşe Gürol and Sevinç Polat

Additional information is available at the end of the chapter

http://dx.doi.org/10.5772/67300

Abstract

Introduction: Children with cancer experience serious difficulties due to the diagnosis, the hospitalization, the symptoms that accompany the long and exhausting treatment process. Unrelieved symptoms related to either cancer or chemotherapy also lead to poorer quality of life, including increased distress and negatively impact healing process. The families of children with cancer often try the complementary and alternative medicine (CAM) to reduce their children's experience of physical discomfort.

Methods: The following sources of published reviews have been consulting: PubMed, The Cochrane Library, and Web of Science. Databases were queried from inception to August 2016. Our inclusion criteria were (i) studies both published in English and between June 1, 2010 and June 31, 2016; (ii) assessment of symptom management and quality of life; and (iii) application of CAM to children with cancer.

Results: In this review, the most commonly used intervention methods were massage, exercise, music and android programs, and yoga, rehabilitation program, art therapy, and reiki therapy. The most commonly evaluated these outcomes: pain, anxiety, fatigue, nausea, sleep, and quality of life in the articles.

Conclusion: National and international collaborations among researchers, policy maker, pharmacist, and clinicians will facilitate the regulated use of effective CAM therapies in pediatric oncology.

Keywords: pediatric oncology, symptoms management, quality of life, evidence-based practices, complementary, alternative medicine

1. Introduction

Cancer and its treatment are stressful, and they reduce the quality of life of cancer patients and their families [1]. Children with cancer experience serious difficulties due to the diagnosis, the hospitalization, the symptoms that accompany the long and exhausting treatment process. As a matter of fact, children with cancer receiving chemotherapy often experience painful conditions such as mucositis and peripheral neuropathy. Unrelieved symptoms related to either cancer or chemotherapy also lead to poorer quality of life, including increased distress and negatively impact healing process [2]. Prevention of symptoms of cancer and side effects of treatment is expected to contribute positively to treatment by increasing the quality of life of children [3].

Children with cancer experience physical symptoms, including pain, and mental symptoms, anxiety [1]. One of these symptoms is also sleeping problems. Sleep disturbances persist in cancer survivors and can cause depression, pain, fatigue, and decrements in quality of life beyond the time of cancer treatment [4, 5]. Sleep problems were often present in a combination of different symptoms [5]. Pain is a common symptom during cancer diagnosis and treatment and may come from painful procedures, disease progression, or impingement of nerves, tissues, or organs from tumors at any stage of the cancer progression [6]. Pain is an unpleasant and subjective experience that involves sensory, affective, cognitive, social, and behavioral components; it is a major cause of human suffering and loss of quality of life [7]. In children and adolescents with cancer, the feeling of fatigue characterized by physical, mental, and emotional components is increasingly observed during and after cancer treatment [8–10]. In addition, many cancer survivors report continued fatigue that adversely impacts their quality of life [8]. Oral mucositis is considered one of the major debilitating side effects of cancer therapy (chemotherapy and radiotherapy). Oral mucositis also impacts on children and adolescents' quality of life and their mood status [11]. Cancer affects to quality of life of children and adolescents with cancer. It has changed their daily physical activities, relationships with their family and friends, emotional well-being, and coping with the symptoms. Throughout this period, pediatric patients suffer from multiple physical and psychological symptoms like pain, fatigue, nausea, to feelings of sadness, worrying, and irritability [12].

The families of children with cancer often try CAM to reduce their children's experience of physical discomfort [1]. Complementary and alternative medicine (CAM), which is not considered as a part of traditional medicine, can be defined as a various medical health care systems, practices, and products. Nowadays, among the most known and applied CAM methods are acupuncture, aromatherapy, osteopathy, yoga, massage, and various herbal supplements [1, 13, 14]. According to the National Center for Complementary and Alternative Medicine (NCCAM), there are three broad categories of CAM: natural products, spiritual care (mind-body), and treatments based on body manipulation [14]. CAMs use in children with cancer has increased worldwide in the last years. The reported frequency of its use varies from 30 to 84% in different surveys [15]. It is important to identify and control symptoms in order to increase quality of life and reduce morbidity. Furthermore, there is some evidence that reduction in symptoms may improve future psychosocial functioning [16].

It has been suggested that the use of CAM, as a component of a healthy lifestyle, may support survivors of childhood cancer in coping with many of these long-term complications and chronic health problems [17]. CAM treatments are mostly used to decrease the side effects of cancer treatment [18, 19].

Complementary and alternative medicine is a method used for supporting the conventional treatment. The main objective in preferring these methods is to increase quality of life and reduce symptoms. CAM therapies have been proven effective for symptoms such as pain, nausea, vomiting, and mucositis [3]. The qualitative and quantitative studies are assessed CAM therapies in these symptom management. But, there is paucity of convincing scientific evidence to support practice of CAM therapies in pediatric cancer patients.

2. Methods

The following sources of published reviews have been consulting: PubMed, The Cochrane Library, and Web of Science. We prepare search filters and consult databases to be accessed. The search strategy used the following subject headings and text words: "complementary and alternative therapy," "pediatric," "cancer," "quality of life," and "symptom." The search was limited to studies including children age zero to 18 years. Databases were queried from inception to August 2016.

Our inclusion criteria were (i) studies both published in English and between June 1, 2010 and June 31, 2016; (ii) assessment of symptom management and quality of life; and (iii) application of CAM to children with cancer.

Articles were excluded at different levels (title, abstract, or full article) based on the following exclusion criteria: all clinical trials published in a language other than English, not published as a full article, animal trials, clinical trials that only involved adults, population not cancer, descriptive studies that were only conducted on the use of complementary therapy and symptoms, case studied and case series, pilot studies, reviews, book chapters, and letters to the editors and commentaries.

The literature investigations were evaluated according to inclusion/exclusion criteria. Then, after a preliminary test, in which their abstract had been searched detailed, the articles were included in the study.

3. Results

Figure 1 illustrates the flow of article selection. A total of 274 articles were identified by the search strategy. Abstracts and titles were initially screened for eligibility. These articles were assessed by the inclusion/exclusion criteria at the different levels of exclusion and yielded a total of 47 articles. Among the 277 articles, 230 (83%) did not meet eligibility criteria. Full text review resulted in 13 articles that were not research studies, 2 articles that included populations other than children and leaving a total of 11 studies included in the review. A total of 20 articles met inclusion criteria and were included in the review (**Table 1**). The articles were published between 2010 and 2016. **Table 1** provides an overview of the studies reviewed, including identified articles, type of intervention, aged group, assessment used measures, and outcomes.

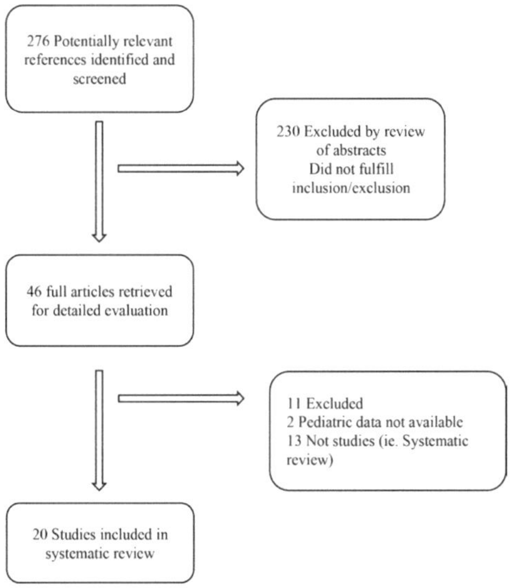

Figure 1. Flow diagram of study identification and selection.

Articles	Aged group	Type of intervention	Outcomes
Barry et al. [22]	11 children and adolescents aged 6–13 years	Music	Distress ↓
Madden et al. [23]	50 children and adolescents aged 2–18 years	Creative art therapy	Pain ↓ Anxiety ↓
Nguyen et al. [24]	40 children and adolescents aged 7–12 years	Music	Pain ↓ Anxiety ↓ Heart rate ↓ Respiratory rate ↓
Yeh et al. [25]	22 children and adolescents aged 0–18 years	Physical exercise	Fatigue ↓
Chamorro-Viña et al. [26]	24 children and adolescents aged 5–18 years	Exercise	Quality of life ↑
Mehling et al. [21]	23 children and adolescents aged 5–18 years	Massage acupressure	Pain ↓ Nausea ↓ Fatigue ↓ Depression ↓ Burden symptom ↓ Anxiety (no change)
da Cunha Batalha and Mota [7]	52 children and adolescents aged 10–18 years	Massage	Pain ↓

Articles	Aged group	Type of intervention	Outcomes
Hooke et al. [20]	29 children and adolescents aged 6–17 years	6-minute walk test	Physical performance (no change)
Tanir and Kuguoglu [27]	40 children and adolescents aged 8–12 years	Exercise program	Pain ↓ Hurt ↓ Nausea ↓ Procedure-related anxiety ↓
Casanova-Garcia et al. [28]	40 children and adolescents aged 5–18 years	GraphPad prism	Neuropathic pain ↓
Çelebioğlu et al. [1]	25 children and adolescents aged 4–15 years	Massage	Anxiety ↓ Pain ↓
Miladinia et al. [29]	43 children and adolescents aged 7–18 years	Massage	Nausea ↓ Frequency of vomit ↓
Beulertz et al. [30]	53 children and adolescents aged 4–17 years	Therapeutic exercise program	Motor performance ↑ Level of activity ↑ Quality of life ↑
Fortier et al. [2]	20 children and adolescents aged 8–18 year	Pain buddy	Pain management ↑
Hooke et al. [31]	13 children and adolescents aged 10–17 years	Yoga	Fatigue ↓ Anxiety ↓ Balance scores ↓ Wellness scores ↓
Hooke et al. [32]	44 children and adolescents aged 6–15 years	Fitness tracker physical activity	Fatigue ↓
Jacobs et al. [4]	45 adolescents aged 12–21 years	Massage	Sleep episodes ↑ Fatigue (no change) Mood (no change) Anxiety (no change) Night time ↑ Overall sleep ↑
Miladinia et al. [33]	35 children and adolescents aged 8–18 years	Slow stroke back massage	Anxiety ↓
Müller et al. [34]	150 children and adolescents aged 4–18 years	Rehabilitation program	Quality of life ↑
Thrane et al. [35]	16 children and adolescents aged 7–16 years	Reiki therapy	Pain ↓ Anxiety ↓ Heart rates ↓ Respiratory rates ↓

Table 1. The effects of complementary and alternative therapy in studies of children and adolescents with cancer.

Characteristics of the 20 articles included in this review are summarized in **Table 1**. The most commonly used intervention methods were massages (six articles), exercise (six articles), music and android programs (every two articles), and yoga, rehabilitation program, art therapy, and reiki therapy (every one article). The most commonly evaluated these outcomes: pain, anxiety, fatigue, nausea, sleep, and quality of life in the articles. However, in some studies [4, 20, 21], CAM utilization was not effective.

4. Discussion

A systematic review of 20 studies of complementary alternative intervention in pediatric oncology patients reported that such interventions are feasible and safe, effects on the symptoms and quality of life. Positive effects were also identified on the pain, sleep, anxiety, nausea, fatigue, quality of life, overall activity levels, and specific aspects of physical function.

It has been reported that the majority of pediatric cancer patients suffer from pain and other symptoms by the World Health Organization. In addition, children with cancer are at high risk for the incidence of symptoms that occur in the treatment process and reduce the quality of their life [2]. Also, whole medical systems are accepted as forms of CAM established on comprehensive systems of theory and practice [36]. Increasingly, parents of children with cancer are requesting the use of CAM therapies on the control of symptoms. CAM therapies increase the patient's and family's feelings of control on their symptoms and develop an understanding of active participation and partnership with the health care provider throughout the healing process [37]. Despite the dozens of pediatric CAM utilization studies, important knowledge gaps continue to persist in this field. CAM is not a static concept and can vary greatly from culture to culture [38]. The decision to use CAM in a child or adolescent with cancer requires consideration of the risks and benefits of the proposed therapy balanced with the developmental needs of the patient and the preferences of the family [39].

CAM consists of four domains, that is (a) mind-body medicine (e.g., meditation, imagery, prayer, art, and music); (b) biologically based practices (e.g., herbs, foods, and vitamins); (c) manipulative and body-based practices (e.g., massage, chiropractic, or osteopathic manipulation); and (d) energy medicine (e.g., Reiki, therapeutic touch, and magnetic fields) [36]. Although this integrative review endeavored to identify all CAM interventions used to manage procedure-related pain, anxiety, distress, and quality of life in children and adolescents undergoing cancer treatment, the only two categories of CAM therapies, manipulative and body-based practices and energy medicine, have been studied in regard to procedure-related symptoms and quality of life in the pediatric oncology population. Of note, other types of CAM therapies, including biologically based therapies (such as herbs, foods, and vitamins), energy therapies (such as acupuncture), and mind-body medicine, have been used for management of nonprocedural cancer-related symptoms (e.g., pain, nausea) and quality of life in children and adolescents with cancer [39]; however, none of these CAM therapies were identified as having been studied in the context of relief of procedure-related symptoms and quality of life in children or adolescents with cancer. Unfortunately, the past 5 years have seen little improvement in the reporting of pediatric CAM utilization data on the children with cancer. Although sample size varied substantially, the largest proportion of studies had ≤50 participants.

Our review had several limitations. In particular, our review includes a focus on pediatric cancer patients, and we only evaluated articles published in the last 5 years, accessed full text articles.

Disclosures and acknowledgements

No funding was received for this review, and there are no financial conflicts of interest associated with this manuscript.

Author details

Ayşe Gürol[1]* and Sevinç Polat[2]*

*Address all correspondence to: ayseparlak42@gmail.com and svnpolat@gmail.com

1 Atatürk University, Health Vocational School, Erzurum, Turkey

2 Bozok University, School of Health, Yozgat, Turkey

References

[1] Çelebioğlu, A., Gürol, A., Yildirim, Z. K., & Büyükavci, M. (2015). Effects of Massage Therapy on Pain and Anxiety Arising from Intrathecal Therapy or Bone Marrow Aspiration in Children with Cancer. International Journal of Nursing Practice, 21(6), 797–804.

[2] Fortier, M. A., Chung, W. W., Martinez, A., Gago-Masague, S., & Sender, L. (2016). Pain Buddy: A Novel Use of M-Health in the Management of Children's Cancer Pain. Computers in Biology and Medicine, 76, 202–214.

[3] Chokshi, S., & Kelly, K. (2012). Potential Role of Complementary and Alternative Medicine in Pediatric Oncology: The Future of CAM Research–Addressing the "Effectiveness Gaps". In: Integrative Pediatric Oncology (pp. 147-156). Springer, Berlin Heidelberg.

[4] Jacobs, S., Mowbray, C., Cates, L. M., Baylor, A., Gable, C., Skora, E., Estrada M., Cheng, Y., Wang, J., Lewin, D., & Hinds, P. (2016). Pilot Study of Massage to Improve Sleep and Fatigue in Hospitalized Adolescents with Cancer. Pediatric Blood Cancer, 63, 880–886.

[5] Walter, L. M., Nixon, G. M., Davey, M. J., Downie, P. A., & Horne, R. S. (2015). Sleep and Fatigue in Pediatric Oncology: A Review of the Literature. Sleep Medicine Reviews, 24, 71–82.

[6] Thrane, S. (2013). Effectiveness of Integrative Modalities for Pain and Anxiety in Children and Adolescents with Cancer A Systematic Review. Journal of Pediatric Oncology Nursing, 30(6), 320–332.

[7] da Cunha Batalha, L. M., & Mota, A. A. (2013). Massage in Children with Cancer: Effectiveness of A Protocol. Jornal de Pediatria, 89(6), 595–600.

[8] Aghabati, N., Mohammadi, E., & Pour Esmaiel, Z. (2010). The Effect of Therapeutic Touch on Pain and Fatigue of Cancer Patients Undergoing Chemotherapy. Evidence-Based Complementary and Alternative Medicine, 7(3), 375–381.

[9] Tomlinson, D., Hinds, P. S., Ethier, M. C., Ness, K. K., Zupanec, S., & Sung, L. (2013). Psychometric Properties of Instruments Used to Measure Fatigue in Children and Adolescents With Cancer: A Systematic Review. Journal of Pain and Symptom Management, 45(1), 83–91.

[10] Tomlinson, D., Diorio, C., Beyene, J., & Sung, L. (2014). Effect of Exercise on Cancer-Related Fatigue: A Meta-Analysis. American Journal of Physical Medicine & Rehabilitation, 93(8), 675–686.

[11] Qutob, A. F., Gue, S., Revesz, T., Logan, R. M., & Keefe, D. (2013). Prevention of Oral Mucositis in Children Receiving Cancer Therapy: A Systematic Review and Evidence-Based Analysis. Oral Oncology, 49(2), 102–107.

[12] Huijer, H. A. S., Sagherian, K., & Tamim, H. (2013). Quality of Life and Symptom Prevalence as Reported by Children with Cancer in Lebanon. European Journal of Oncology Nursing, 17(6), 704–710.

[13] Bishop, F. L., Prescott, P., Chan, Y. K., Saville, J., von Elm, E., & Lewith, G. T. (2010). Prevalence of Complementary Medicine Use in Pediatric Cancer: A Systematic Review. Pediatrics, 125(4), 768–776.

[14] Poder, T. G., & Lemieux, R. (2014). How Effective Are Spiritual Care and Body Manipulation Therapies in Pediatric Oncology? A Systematic Review of the Literature. Global Journal of Health Science, 6(2), 112.

[15] Turhan, A. B., & Bör, Ö. (2016). Use of Herbs or Vitamin/Mineral/Nutrient Supplements by Pediatric Oncology Patients. Complementary Therapies in Clinical Practice, 23, 69–74.

[16] Dupuis, L. L., Ethier, M. C., Tomlinson, D., Hesser, T., & Sung, L. (2012). A Systematic Review of Symptom Assessment Scales in Children with Cancer. BMC Cancer, 12(1), 430.

[17] Ndao, D. H., Ladas, E. J., Bao, Y., Cheng, B., Nees, S. N., Levine, J. M., & Kelly, K. M. (2013). Use of Complementary and Alternative Medicine Among Children, Adolescent, and Young Adult Cancer Survivors: A Survey Study. Journal of Pediatric Hematology/Oncology, 35(4), 281–288.

[18] Adams, D., Spelliscy, C., Sivakumar, L., Grundy, P., Leis, A., Sencer, S., & Vohra, S. (2013). CAM and Pediatric Oncology: Where Are All The Best Cases?. Evidence-Based Complementary and Alternative Medicine, 2013, 6 p.

[19] Karalı, Y., Demirkaya, M., & Sevinir, B. (2012). Use of Complementary and Alternative Medicine in Children with Cancer: Effect on Survival. Pediatric Hematology and Oncology, 29(4), 335–344.

[20] Hooke, M. C., Garwick, A. W., & Neglia, J. P. (2013). Assessment of Physical Performance Using the 6-Minute Walk Test in Children Receiving Treatment for Cancer. Cancer Nursing, 36(5), E9–E16.

[21] Mehling, W. E., Lown, E. A., Dvorak, C. C., Cowan, M. J., Horn, B. N., Dunn, E. A., Acree M., Abrams D. I., & Hecht, F. M. (2012). Hematopoietic Cell Transplant and Use of Massage for Improved Symptom Management: Results from A Pilot Randomized Control Trial. Evidence-Based Complementary and Alternative Medicine, 2012, 450150.

[22] Barry, P., O'Callaghan, C., Wheeler, G., Grocke, D. (2010). Music Therapy CD Creation for Initial Pediatric Radiation Therapy: A Mixed Methods Analysis. Journal of Music Therapy, 47(3), 233–263.

[23] Madden, J. R., Mowry, P., Gao, D., Cullen, P. M., & Foreman, N. K. (2010). Creative Arts Therapy Improves Quality of Life for Pediatric Brain Tumor Patients Receiving Outpatient Chemotherapy. Journal of Pediatric Oncology Nursing, 27(3), 133–145.

[24] Nguyen, T. N., Nilsson, S., Hellström, A. L., & Bengtson, A. (2010). Music Therapy to Reduce Pain and Anxiety in Children With Cancer Undergoing Lumbar Puncture: A Randomized Clinical Trial. Journal of Pediatric Oncology Nursing, 27(3), 146–155.

[25] Yeh, C. H., Wai, J. P. M., Lin, U. S., & Chiang, Y. C. (2011). A Pilot Study to Examine the Feasibility and Effects of A Home-Based Aerobic Program on Reducing Fatigue in Children With Acute Lymphoblastic Leukemia. Cancer Nursing, 34(1), 3–12.

[26] Chamorro-Viña, C., Guilcher, G. M., Khan, F. M., Mazil, K., Schulte, F., Wurz, A., Williamson T., Reimer R. A., & Culos-Reed, S. N. (2012). EXERCISE in Pediatric Autologous Stem Cell Transplant Patients: A Randomized Controlled Trial Protocol. BMC Cancer, 12(1), 401.

[27] Tanir, M. K., & Kuguoglu, S. (2013). Impact of Exercise on Lower Activity Levels in Children with Acute Lymphoblastic Leukemia: A Randomized Controlled Trial from Turkey. Rehabilitation Nursing, 38(1), 48–59.

[28] Casanova-García, C., Lara, S. L., Ruiz, M. P., Domínguez, D. R., & Sosa, E. S. (2015). Non-pharmacological Treatment for Neuropathic Pain in Children with Cancer. Medical Hypotheses, 85(6), 791–797.

[29] Miladinia, M., Baraz, S., Mousavi Nouri, E., & Gholamzadeh Baeis, M. (2015). Effects of Slow-Stroke Back Massage on Chemotherapy-induced Nausea and Vomiting in the Pediatrics with Acute Leukemia: A Challenge of Controlling Symptoms. International Journal of Pediatrics, 3(6.2), 1145–1152.

[30] Beulertz, J., Prokop, A., Rustler, V., Bloch, W., Felsch, M., & Baumann, F. T. (2016). Effects of a 6-Month, Group-Based, Therapeutic Exercise Program for Childhood Cancer Outpatients on Motor Performance, Level of Activity, and Quality of Life. Pediatric Blood & Cancer, 63(1), 127–132.

[31] Hooke, M. C., Gilchrist, L., Foster, L., Langevin, M., & Lee, J. (2016a). Yoga for Children and Adolescents After Completing Cancer Treatment. Journal of Pediatric Oncology Nursing, 33(1), 64–73.

[32] Hooke, M. C., Gilchrist, L., Tanner, L., Hart, N., & Withycombe, J. S. (2016b). Use of a Fitness Tracker to Promote Physical Activity in Children with Acute Lymphoblastic Leukemia. Pediatric Blood & Cancer, 63(4), 684–689.

[33] Miladinia, M., Fakharzadeh, L., Zarea, K., & Mousavi Nouri, E. (2016). Anxiety Control in the Iranian Children with Chronic Leukemia: Use of a Non-drug Method. International Journal of Pediatrics, 4(1), 1225–1231.

[34] Müller, C., Krauth, K. A., Gerß, J., & Rosenbaum, D. (2016). Physical Activity and Health-Related Quality of Life in Pediatric Cancer Patients Following A 4-Week Inpatient Rehabilitation Program. Supportive Care in Cancer, 24:3793–3802.

[35] Susan E. Thrane, Scott H. Maurer, Dianxu Ren, Cynthia A. Danford, Susan M. Cohen. Reiki Therapy for Symptom Management in Children Receiving Palliative Care A Pilot Study. American Journal Hospice and Palliative Medicine, (First Published 10 Jul 2016), February 7, 2016, http://journals.sagepub.com/doi/full/10.1177/1049909116630973.

[36] NCCAM. CAM Basics. 2007. Retrieved April 21, 2009, from http://nccam.nih.gov/health/whatiscam/overview.htm.

[37] Sencer, S. F., & Kelly, K. M. (2007). Complementary and Alternative Therapies in Pediatric Oncology. Pediatric Clinics of North America, 54(6), 1043–1060.

[38] Surette, S., Vanderjagt, L., & Vohra, S. (2013). Surveys of Complementary and Alternative Medicine Usage: A Scoping Study of the Paediatric Literature. Complementary Therapies in Medicine, 21, S48–S53.

[39] Landier, W., & Alice, M. T. (2010). Use of Complementary and Alternative Medical Interventions for The Management of Procedure-Related Pain, Anxiety, and Distress in Pediatric Oncology: An Integrative Review. Journal of Pediatric Nursing, 25(6), 566–579.

Chapter 4

The Forgotten Children

Christopher Kuo and Paul M. Kent

Additional information is available at the end of the chapter

http://dx.doi.org/10.5772/67042

Abstract

The "forgotten children" of pediatric cancer are the siblings. There is a dearth of literature published on the effects of cancer on the siblings' psychosocial state. Despite significant improvements made in the survival of pediatric cancer patients, the psychosocial health of the siblings remains the same. The siblings' need for support and understanding continue to go unnoticed. The aim of this chapter is to shed light on the roles siblings play in the pediatric cancer trajectory, as well as to recognize the emotional and psychological toll they endure through the experience of diagnosis, treatment, survival, and bereavement as the "forgotten children."

Keywords: forgotten children, siblings of children with cancer, pediatric cancer, psychosocial, siblings cancer trajectory

1. Introduction

"I was the one that had to convince my parents to let Stanley stop all curative treatment. It was traumatic. To feel like you're giving up, but obligated to do what your dying brother asks, and to realize that his time was up. It wasn't the palliative service or his primary oncologist's job to do it. It was my job. I was the only one that could get through to our parents, and 'til this day I still remember… telling our parents that it's time to let go."

The three common themes of siblings of childhood cancer include changing lives, intense feelings, and unmet needs [1]. The sibling bond is one of the most powerful and lengthy connections across a lifetime [2]. It is a source of unconditional love mixed with rivalry. Siblings shape each other's identity. Thus, understanding how pediatric cancer can affect healthy siblings is fundamental to the patient's psychosocial care. The siblings of children with cancer are often missed or neglected and known as the "forgotten children" [3–5].

In the late 1980s, the emotional disorders in siblings of children with chronic illnesses were a new focus in the literature [4]. Following these studies were reports focusing specifically on siblings of pediatric cancer patients. Carpenter et al. [6] designed one of the earlier studies to utilize camping programs to address and investigate how siblings of children with cancer were feeling. In 1999, guidelines were established by the International Society of Pediatric Oncology (SIOP) working committee on psychosocial issues in pediatric oncology to provide assistance to siblings of children with cancer [7]. The guidelines addressed different domains of cancer trajectory such as diagnosis, treatment, relapse, and completion of treatment. The authors hoped to involve siblings of children with cancer throughout their siblings' experiences with cancer [7]. However, two decades later, many of these issues they sought to address, such as the feelings of isolation, lack of involvement, and lack of understanding, continue to exist [2].

Pediatric cancer is a disparate illness experience from adult cancer and elicits different approaches in families. The burdens of pediatric cancer include the long-term psychosocial effects, compromised social well-being on the child and the family, chronic medical conditions, and the mental and financial drain upon the families [8]. The initial diagnosis of childhood cancer brings a significant level of distress to the entire family, with the death of a child as the most traumatic experience a family suffers [2].

Caring for a child with cancer is extremely demanding and stressful. Due to the intimate and personal emotional connections of family caregivers, the burdens they face are unequivocally different than those faced by pediatric oncologists or the patient. In addition, family caregivers often unconsciously share the unyielding burden of cancer with the ill child. Throughout treatment, the focus inevitably is on the ill child, leaving the siblings in a vulnerable position [2]. Published literature remains scarce on the psychosocial distress of siblings. These circumstances highlight the need to address pediatric cancer through the siblings' perspective.

2. Body

2.1. Diagnosis

"*Seeing him there made me think, 'Why is it him? Why is it not me?'* [9]."

From the moment the diagnosis is given, until their death, siblings of children with cancer are unmoored. Cancer affects patients and families both emotionally and physically [10]. From the time of diagnosis to treatment, survivorship, recurrence, and palliation, the incidence of patient's emotional distress ranges from 35% to 45% [11–13]. Psychological distress has become the "sixth vital sign" in cancer care; however, there is little existing research focusing on the "sixth vital sign" of the siblings [10].

Family dynamic is always disrupted when a child is diagnosed with cancer. During diagnosis, families are hurled into chaos and haunted by complex medical language, life-or-death decisions, and emergency admissions of unknown duration [8]. Parents face loss of employment, divorce/separation, relocation of home, and often decide not to have more children [14]. Siblings

http://dx.doi.org/10.5772/67042

become overwhelmed with the lack of support and burden of the unknown. Regardless of age, siblings are often forced to take on roles that exceed their maturity level. They are expected to take on adult responsibilities and decision-making roles, such as caring for the family, becoming financially independent, and making informed medical decisions for the ill sibling [15]. Siblings may also act as the mediator between parents who may disagree about treatment or otherwise face marital difficulties. Ultimately, these myriad roles may lead to intrusive thoughts and conflicting emotions such as anger, jealousy, fear, loneliness, or guilt [16].

"It was exhausting, to say the least, to try to live a normal life. To continue to go to my classes pretending that everything was okay, while deep down inside everything was crumbling apart. Stanley just got diagnosed with cancer. I had to make sure my parents were mentally and emotionally stable. I had to make sure I was there for Stanley, my parents and my younger brother. I was trying my best to hold everything together. Ironically, everything was falling apart, yet no one could tell from the outside."

2.1.1. Isolation

The "forgotten children" are isolated from support systems both inside and outside the family [3–5]. The siblings may become self-centered, lonely, and envious of diverted parental attention. Their distress stems from the changes in family dynamics and routine; concerns over the cause and outcome of the illness; observing their sibling's suffering; and feelings of unworthiness, guilt, anger, sadness, and rejection [17–21]. Compared with siblings of children with other chronic illnesses, siblings of children with cancer endure more emotional distress and adaptive difficulties [22].

The difference between patient and caregiver psychological distress varies over time [23]. There is significantly more distress on the caregiver when the patient is receiving treatment initially. However, 1–2 months after initiating treatment, patients report more distress than their caregivers [23]. During their treatment course, siblings experience progressive physical and emotional demands, while the healthcare team tends to the patient. However, as time progresses, the psychological distress between the patient and the siblings becomes the same. SIOP recommends that early intervention with siblings should be implemented to prevent the initial development of psychological distress [7, 23].

"I remember Stanley was brought to the ED once due to shortness of breath. I got a call from my mom yelling that I need to be there immediately. That night felt like an eternity. I thought he was going to die. I didn't want to let him go, and I wasn't ready. It happened so quickly. Ever since then, I worry if every day is the last day for him."

The lack of attention to the siblings is shown in the discrepancy between survivor-parent and sibling-parent reports of health-related quality of life (HRQL) [24]. Survivors reported higher HRQL than parent-proxy reports, whereas siblings reported lower HRQL than parent-proxy reports, suggesting that parents often see their child who survived cancer as doing worse than their child without a history of cancer, although both the survivor and sibling report similar HRQL [24]. This discrepancy between parents' report and siblings' own report of their physical, emotion, and social well-being reflects on the inherent parental bias that siblings are always "fine," thereby requiring less attention than their sick child [24].

Children need to develop competencies across a number of areas as they grow. Yet siblings of children with cancer are often limited to their engagement in daily activities, such as leisure and peer relationships. Infants and toddlers are most at risk for behavioral or emotional problems as they interpret the changes in the family as rejection [25]. Many younger siblings (age, 7–11) have impaired emotional/social and decreased quality of life even 2 years after the cancer diagnosis. Others have reported that adolescent siblings appear to be more at risk for adjustment difficulties [26].

Guggemos et al. [27] compared 14 siblings of children diagnosed with cancer with matched control group of 18 children age 6–12 and discovered that 2 weeks after the cancer diagnosis, siblings of children with cancer displayed more guilt or shame, avoided displaying interpersonal conflicts, showed problems of dysregulation, and had significantly more elements of disruptions, destruction and themes of dissociation. The well siblings have a tendency to manipulate and control the situation and the interviewer by changing the rules of play, which reflects their confusion and fear of losing control over the course of the story [27]. It is suggested that shortly after diagnosis, siblings showed clear reactions of intrapsychic adjustment that may be prognostic for the later development of mental illness [27]. All siblings described a sense of shock, fear, uncertainty, and loneliness following the diagnosis of cancer [9].

"*I started drinking and partying but never got in trouble. I would be blackout drunk and driving home… So there, I think, I wanted somebody to ask me, 'How are you doing?' but nobody ever did* [15]."

2.2. Treatment phase

Through being a sibling-caregiver, siblings have been reported to develop unique ways of being in the world, consisting of three themes revolving around the family: committing to keeping the family together, being present, and enduring sadness [28]. One of the most common experiences that siblings have during treatment is the disintegration of their normal life routine. The continual shift of family's focus to the child with cancer forces the healthy siblings to experience chaos and disorder in their personal and family life [29].

During the treatment phase, siblings often undergo an emotional roller coaster, experiencing a mixture of positive and negative emotions: the initial feelings of fear and uncertainty continue to linger, their lives revolve around their siblings' suffering, and family life remains in limbo [9].

"*Her [warning sign] is temperatures and infections. We always have a bag packed. We are always prepared to leave* [9]."

"*I don't plan anything; I don't; I haven't for years. We go from day to day- that's the only way I can make it work. If I plan for anything further than 2–3 days in advance, it doesn't work. It never seems to work, and I just don't bother anymore* [30]."

During treatment, siblings often have inadequate information about details of the cancer. The family may withhold information due to concerns of sibling's young age and their own limited understanding [29]. Younger siblings (6–10 years old) might not comprehend the gravity of the disease until they witness the alopecia, fatigue, weight loss, and other physical changes of their siblings [29]. These siblings can be emotionally trapped, and their peers are too young or naïve to understand cancer and death. Eventually, the siblings cultivate inexpressible sentiments, and end up internalizing the negative emotions.

A study by Prchal and Landolt. [31] showed that at school, siblings are frequently bombarded with questions regarding the ill child's condition and diagnosis from their teachers and classmates. Siblings ultimately preferred to volunteer the information about their ill sibling's condition instead of being forced to report. Many siblings put up a facade of normalcy to avoid discussing their sibling's condition and to avoid pity, which may make them uncomfortable.

"*Well, everyone at school came to me and asked how my brother was doing. Even the teachers kept asking. And after a while I thought, why do they always have to come and ask me?* [31]"

"*Eventually, I started lying to the question 'how many siblings do you have?' just to avoid discussing the fact that my brother has cancer. I hate that question and I hate having to talk about Stanley's cancer. I hate anticipating the sympathetic stares just because Stanley has cancer. Not a lot of people knew Stanley had cancer. I was living a double life.*"

Older siblings (11–18 years old) may be able to look after their brother or sister with sympathy [29]. However, they may also experience learning difficulties at school and have diminished peer interactions [29]. Siblings may also experience a mix of empathy, worry, anger, jealousy, and a loss of self-esteem [29]. Despite these difficulties, several studies have shown that the "forgotten children" may transcend the chaos [29], reporting strengthened relationships with their ill brother/sister, deep appreciation for time spent together, a desire to do more together whenever possible, and they continue to uphold a positive attitude when assisting with family matters [9, 29]. Siblings become more mature and sensible, independent, and able to help with family routines and household duties [29]. They develop an impeccable sense of resilience, sympathy, and love for others [29]. Many siblings reconstruct their roles as the sick brother's or sister's protector, constantly facing unpleasant situations with an optimistic outlook and making efforts to reconstruct the family order [29]. They learn that "being present" was essential to their peace of mind [28]. They balance solitude and abandonment with a need for belonging and intimacy in the family [29]. Maintaining family cohesiveness becomes the focus during the treatment phase.

2.3. Survivorship

With improved survival, late adverse outcomes of treatment have become more prevalent, posing a new challenge for the family caregivers [32]. As patients gradually transition into survivorship, the roles and demands of caregivers change [33]. The early transition can be uncertain and overwhelm families with a sense of uncertainty about the future [33]. The family may ruminate on the thought of recurrence or a secondary malignancy. Unfortunately, studies on sibling caregivers in these transitional periods have not been done.

During the course of cancer, siblings center activities around their ill sibling. They relinquish valued personal activities, relationships, and opportunities. Once treatment is over, some siblings have an extremely difficult time restoring normalcy. Past relationships may no longer exist; friends, social support, and opportunities may have moved on [33]. Siblings have a strong desire to reintegrate back to a normal life but often end up establishing a new normal instead.

In contrast to the transition period, studies have been done on sibling caregivers after treatment completion. In 2015, Guggemos et al. [27] reported that siblings of children with cancer at the end of treatment continue to display dysregulative behaviors and continue to remain at risk. Several studies have reported that siblings of young cancer survivors have more negative psychological distress (e.g., fear, worry, anger), more posttraumatic stress, and poorer quality of life compared to controls [34, 35]. In contrast, a 1995 study of 60 siblings of cancer survivors measuring psychosocial adjustment found that after treatment, siblings adjusted well with no major differences in psychosocial functioning compared to peers with healthy siblings [4, 36, 37]. They hypothesized that after treatment, siblings are able to distance themselves from the cancer experience, whereas survivors continue to confront the disease [4].

2.3.1. Posttraumatic growth

It has been theorized that after the traumatic experience with cancer, individuals will achieve posttraumatic growth (PTG). PTG is defined as developing resilience from a previous trauma, perceiving benefits from it and developing beyond the original level of psychological functioning [38]. Siblings have been reported to experience less PTG than parents but did experience similar levels of PTG to the survivors [39]. Older siblings were found to utilize more active coping strategies such as actively seeking social support [39]. The longer it had been since the original cancer diagnosis, the less avoidant coping strategies and more positive life satisfaction were present [39]. PTG after cancer experience stimulates the development of five themes, making sense of cancer experience, appreciation of life, greater self-knowledge, positive attitude toward family, and a desire to pay back society [40]. The experience of being a part of their siblings' cancer experience triggers an existential challenge of life, which leads to a search for meaning or purpose to life. Ultimately, siblings may make up their own meaning in order to resolve or make sense of the tragedy [40]. They may live by the carpe diem philosophy, living more consciously and able to put things in perspective [40]. Currently, more studies are needed to establish a general consensus on the psychological effects of siblings during the survival stage.

2.4. Bereavement

Although the survival of childhood cancer has approached near 80% due to treatment advances [41], many cancers remain terminal at the time of diagnosis (i.e., intrinsic pontine glioma), or the state of science has stagnated for decades with no increase in survival (i.e., osteosarcoma) [8]. Many of the patients ultimately succumb. The cancer journey initially begins with the hope for cure or remission. Yet the optimism often plateaus as the families eventually realize that the hope may become one for a comfortable ending [8].

2.4.1. Communication

Studies have shown very poor communication with siblings regarding the death of their brother/sister. In the last 24 hours before the loss, 43% of the siblings reported getting no information about the impending death of their siblings from a family member, while 70% were not informed by one of the healthcare professionals [42]. Additionally, it was not until

<24 hours before their brother's/sister's death that the sibling understood their death intellectually (53%) and emotionally (76%) [42]. Eighty-four percent reported that nobody talked to them about what to expect when their brother/sister was dying, and these siblings showed significantly higher levels of anxiety up to 9 years later compared with those who knew what to expect [42]. More than one-fourth did not want to discuss their siblings' death, while one-third wished they had talked more with their families about it [33]. Cancer-bereaved siblings report lower self-esteem, sleep disturbances, and lower levels of maturity 2–9 years after the sibling's loss in comparison with non-bereaved siblings [43]. A nationwide survey in Sweden exploring siblings' experiences of their brother's/sister's cancer death found persistent levels of anxiety 2–9 years later [42].

2.4.2. Death aftermath

During the time of death, some siblings described that death came so rapidly that they weren't able to be there [42]. Those that were present at the time of death expressed gratitude and closure, including a sense of relief as death alleviated further suffering [42]. Shortly after death, however, some siblings felt emptiness and guilt that they were the ones still alive [42].

Siblings 12 years bereaved (mean age of 26 years) reported higher illegal drug and alcohol use during the year immediately after their sibling's death than before their sibling's diagnosis but then eventually returned to baseline [44]. Additionally, a similar trajectory was observed with anxiety and depression scores consistent with high distress in those who were unprepared for their sibling's death, unable to say goodbye and had not worked through their grief [44]. Twelve years later, 88% of respondents reported that the loss of sibling continued to affect their daily lives, 12% negatively, 45% positively, and impacted their education and career choices [44]. Although the majority of bereaved siblings have not worked through their grief, most siblings ultimately recover from the cancer experience without residual psychological distress [45].

van der Geest et al. [46] studied parental perceptions of bereaved sibling's well-being. They found that 43% of parents reported that siblings at home experienced a lot of distress in the period immediately before and after the death of the sibling and 46% reported continued negative consequences even after 5 years [46]. This correlates to Rosenberg et al.'s [44] report that during the immediate period surrounding loss, siblings experience severe emotional trauma, but majority ultimately normalize after 12 years.

Time, communication, and consistent support during the bereavement phase may allow siblings to heal. Furthermore, equivalent to PTG in survival stage, positive outcomes upon bereavement were also reported, such as better communication (36%), more maturity (43%), more kindness (45%), and more confidence than peers in their age (17%) [44].

2.5. Interventions/support

Since 1999, guidelines have been established to address siblings' needs; however, many of the recommendations relied on the parents, and on supportive services, which typically are not established in the hospital system (psychosocial support programs, sibling support group, and parent support groups), which make these guidelines unrealistic [7]. Interestingly, majority of the published perspectives on siblings are through pediatric oncology nursing journals, and pediatric oncology nurses often rate the utility of psychosocial screening tools higher than pediatric oncologists and social workers [47]. In 2005, the National Institute for Health and Clinical Excellence (NICE) in the United Kingdom developed guidance for healthcare professions to address siblings of children with cancer [48]. NICE suggested structured psychosocial assessment at significant time points throughout the cancer trajectory such as at diagnosis, treatment, relapse, and bereavement [48]. Although NICE guidelines are helpful, it is unknown if they are being utilized. The NICE guidelines parallel a report from the Institute of Medicine in the United States, which emphasized that the efforts to improve biopsychosocial health of children with cancer should be extended to members of their family [49]. Between 1990 and 2012, various organizations attempted to create standards, guidelines, and consensus reports regarding pediatric psycho-oncology care (**Tables 1–3**). However, rarely do these published reports specifically address siblings as a separate entity from "family" Of children with cancer, even though there is an understanding that siblings have a unique cancer experience. Additionally, between 1990 and 2009, publications on the experiences of siblings of children with cancer grew dramatically [34]. Various qualitative and quantitative studies have been published, but little has changed since these reports. Siblings continue to be the "forgotten children" in the family, and their needs remain unmet.

Currently, there is no standardized tool designed for healthcare professionals (HCPs) to screen for psychosocial needs in pediatric cancer [50]. Available comprehensive screening tools are listed in **Table 4**. Psychosocial Care Checklist (PCCL) is a tool developed to address this gap [51]. The results indicated that oncologists and nurses do not seem to have the same awareness of psychosocial problems in the family compared to the social workers [50].

2.5.1. Intervention

One of the earliest interventions developed for siblings of children with cancer was peer support camp [6]. Camp as a therapeutic intervention has been utilized in various chronic diseases such as diabetes, asthma, renal disease, and cancer. However, camps in pediatric oncology have mainly focused on the child with cancer and rarely on the "forgotten children." Although camps for siblings do exist, the majority of them are for bereaved siblings [52]. Sidhu et al. [2] developed therapeutic peer support camp as an intervention for siblings of 8–13 years of children with cancer on active treatment. Siblings who attended the camp reported lower levels of distress, decreased isolation, decreased anxiety, improved social competence, and greater social acceptance [2]. Through camp, siblings had significant reduction in the fear of cancer, manifested through improved knowledge of cancer and its treatment [2].

2.5.2. What siblings want

Lovgren et al. [53] conducted a nationwide survey of bereaved siblings answering open-ended question about what advice they would give to healthcare professionals (HCPs) working with pediatric cancer patients and their families. The commonly reported advice was related to the siblings' wish for support regardless of their age [53]. They wanted insight into their own feelings in relation to their family and information about their sibling's disease and care [53]. Siblings also wished for support groups, activities, someone to talk to, and asked HCP to not give up trying to offer help [53]. Surprisingly, the "little things" were just as meaningful, such as when HCPs offered them a game, a sticker, a snack, or a hug [53].

Year published	Standard established by	What did it address?	Did it address specifically to siblings?	Reference
1996	ASPHO Health Care Reform and Public Issues Committee	Rationale and recommendations for a comprehensive pediatric hematology/oncology program to be implemented throughout the disease trajectory with services of psychosocial personnel explicitly described	No	[61]
2002	International Society of Pediatric Oncology (SIOP)	Standards for care of children with cancer that proposed ideal care	No	[62]
2008	US Institute of Medicine	*Cancer Care for the Whole Patient: Meeting Psychosocial Health Needs*	Minimal recommendations addressed specifically to siblings of children with cancer, e.g., "primary and other HCPs should monitor caregivers, children, and *siblings* of survivors for signs of psychological distress both during the survivor's treatment and in the post-treatment period. Cancer care providers should inform families of cancer patients about supportive services, including special camps for families and *siblings*	[63]
2010	Canadian Association of Psychosocial Oncology (CAPO)	"Standards of psychosocial health services for person with cancer and their families."—Developed to assist cancer facilities, administrators, program leaders, and professionals in the delivery of psychosocial heath services in Canada by providing a basic framework for these services	No, addressed "family" but never directly addressed siblings	[64]
2013	The European Society of Pediatric Oncology	European Standards of Care for Children with Cancer	No, addressed "family" but never directly addressed siblings	[65]

Table 1. Published standards addressing pediatric cancer population.

Year published	Guidelines established by	What did it address?	Did it address specifically to siblings?	Reference
1999	International Society of Pediatric Oncology (SIOP)	Guidelines for assistance to siblings of children with cancer	Yes	[7]
2000	Researchers at the University of Bonn	Structuring psychosocial care in pediatric oncology—oriented to specific phases of medical treatment of pediatric cancer patients, specifically focusing on the importance of multidisciplinary teams and the role of psychosocial professionals	No, addressed family as a whole and discussed family-oriented care, but never directly addressed siblings	[66]
2005	National Institute for Health and Clinical Excellence (NICE)	Improving outcomes in children and young people with cancer	Yes, addressed siblings but still focused mainly on the family	[48]
2012	National Comprehensive Cancer Network (NCCN)	Guidelines published for the support of adolescents and young adults living with cancer and their families	No, addressed family as a whole and discussed family-oriented care, but never directly addressed siblings	[67]

Table 2. Published guidelines addressing pediatric cancer population.

Information regarding the disease is often intentionally left out to the siblings by parents or HCP. Yet siblings felt that information should be given continuously by the HCPs during treatment, progression, and prognosis [53]. Siblings pointed out that their own needs for information often differed from those of their parents and they had a right to be given information that their parents refused to take in [53]. It was important for HCPs to remain realistic and honest, focus on the bright moments, and promote happiness and hope even during times of suffering [53].

Since 2013, "sibling supporters" have been available to provide support to siblings at six pediatric oncology units in Sweden [54]. They are resource persons whose main task is to see the siblings of those who become sick [54]. They participate in various activities together, listen to their narratives, and are present during the time of illness, survivorship, and bereavement [54]. They facilitated opportunities for similar siblings to meet each other, to discuss things that a sibling was unable to say or understand, and to facilitate conversations with parents and professionals [54]. They were also able to remain positive and create outings for siblings outside the hospital that disassociate them from sickness and death [54].

"*In the hospital, there wasn't really anywhere for siblings to go…I think there needs to be a [designated] place for siblings to go, people for them to talk to* [9]."

Siblings are exceptionally vulnerable to Post-Traumatic Stress Disorder (PTSD) during the initial months after diagnosis [44, 46]: in the first 2 months, 23% and 43% of siblings have full and partial DSM-IV PTSD, respectively [16, 44, 46]. With early psychological intervention,

Year published	Consensus statements established by	What did it address?	Did it address specifically to siblings?	Reference
1998	American Federation of Clinical Oncologic Societies	Consensus statement on providing access to quality cancer care—focused on medical treatment and intervention and offered recommendations for support groups, counseling services, and professional psychotherapeutic services	No, focused primarily on the patient	[68]
2004	NCCN	Evidence-based consensus statement regarding the care and support needs of children and young people with leukemia and their families	Yes, a minor chapter on sibling support that consists of one paragraph: "Appropriate support for siblings is crucial. As with parents, this should encompass easily accessible, age appropriate and honest information and opportunities for siblings to discuss their feelings and fears." Additionally, addressed siblings as a separate entity throughout the consensus document	[69]
2010	LIVESTRONG Young Adult Alliance	Recommendations for quality cancer care for adolescents and young adults—identified four critical elements of quality care, access to healthcare professionals, treatment and medical intervention, and psychosocial support	No, focused primarily on the patient and did not address family or siblings	[70]

Table 3. Published consensus addressing pediatric cancer population.

Screening tools	Function	References
Health-related quality of life (HRQL)	Multidimensional construct that encompasses the physical, psychological, and social domains of functioning	[71]
Psychosocial Care Checklist (PCCL)	Instrument developed to assist HCPs to identify psychosocial issues for a child with cancer and his/her family	[50]
Distress thermometer	Assesses general distress using a thermometer-like scale varying from 0 to 10	[72]
Psychosocial assessment tool (PAT) and PAT 2.0	Family-focused instrument designed to be completed by a parent and screens for psychosocial risk factors associated with childhood cancer	[73, 74]

Table 4. Comprehensive screening tools for siblings of children with cancer.

siblings reported better psychosocial well-being, better medical knowledge and better social support, but no statistical correlation with acute anxiety or PTSD [16].

Open age-appropriate communications with siblings regarding the possibility of the ill child dying and giving them a chance to say goodbye can provide comfort and closure. Serious psychological issues are rare with the involvement of palliative care [55]. Siblings need guidance on what to expect [29].

"*The moment it came out [diagnosis], I could only think of the fact that my brother could die* [31]."

"*He was [unreasonably] demanding. Sometimes he wanted sausages with ketchup and all sorts of things at 1 o'clock in the morning, and during a certain phase, he got aggressive very fast* [31]."

Bereavement follow-up after the death of a child has been recommended as a standard of care in pediatric oncology [56]. Lichtenthal et al. [56] recommend that a member of the healthcare team should contact the family after a child's death to assess family needs, to identify those at risk for negative psychosocial sequelae, to continue care, and to provide resources for bereavement support. It has been suggested that pediatric palliative care clinicians have an ethical duty of "nonabandonment," to care for the families of children with life-threatening conditions through their illness and times of bereavement [57]. Perhaps, these recommendations should be adopted for the siblings of children with cancer also.

A standard of care for siblings of children with cancer should also be established [58]. Parents and professionals should be advised about tools and therapies to meet siblings' unmet needs (**Table 4**) [58]. These should include psychoeducation, coping and prevention strategies, as well as assessment and treatment of psychopathology spanning diagnosis to bereavement[58].

3. Conclusions

The scope of medical care for pediatric oncology should extend beyond the control of cancer to the psychosocial care of the child and siblings' family [50]. Standard guidelines, established since the 1990s [7, 48, 49], are rarely implemented as the standard of care. Barriers from implementing them include predisposing factors, enabling factors, and reinforcing factors (**Table 5**) [59].

Barriers	Examples
Predisposing factors	Lack of knowledge, training, beliefs and attitudes, self efficacy
Enabling factors	Lack of consultation time, assessment skills and systems, skills to intervene, role definition
Reinforcing factors	Lack of feedback, rewards, negative consequences

Table 5. Barriers for pediatric oncologists in implementing psychosocial communication.

In North America's pediatric cancer centers, early psychosocial screening is neither consistently nor systematically conducted and/or documented [60]. It is imperative that physicians are aware of the psychosocial issues that exist within the family, as these issues could identify critical factors that may affect the medical treatment and family cohesiveness [50]. PCCL is a promising screening tool that could assist with enhancing HCPs' awareness of the psychosocial issues for the child with cancer and his/her family [50].

Siblings endure various distresses throughout the different stages of cancer trajectory. Although their voices are gradually being heard, the complexity of the roots of their distress requires meticulous attention to dissect and unravel. The goal is to ultimately have a supportive and therapeutic system in place to assist the siblings during their times of distress.

Research on the psychosocial well-being for siblings of children with cancer remains limited. Consistencies with screening and supportive interventions continue to be lacking. A standardized screening tool with early interventional services should be implemented, such as PCCL and sibling supportive camps. Additionally, interdisciplinary awareness of the siblings' psychosocial issues should be increased in order to shed light to their invisibility. The goal is to remember the "forgotten children."

Acknowledgements

In loving memory of Stanley Kuo and Sammy Kuo, this chapter is dedicated to Cody Kuo, Amy Chen, Peggy Chen, Angel Chiang, and all the siblings affected by cancer. Special thanks to Jeff Ording.

Author details

Christopher Kuo[1] and Paul M. Kent[2*]

*Address all correspondence to: paul_kent@rush.edu

1 Rush Medical College, Chicago, IL, United States

2 Division of Pediatric Hematology/Oncology, Department of Pediatrics, Rush University Medical Center, Chicago, IL, United States

References

[1] Wilkins KL, Woodgate RL. A review of qualitative research on the childhood cancer experience from the perspective of siblings: a need to give them a voice. J Pediatr Oncol Nurs. 2005 Nov–Dec;22(6):305–319.

[2] Sidhu, R, Passmore, A and Baker, D. The effectiveness of a peer support camp for siblings of children with cancer. Pediatr Blood Cancer. (2006);47: 580–588. doi:10.1002/pbc.20653

[3] Massimo LM, Wiley TJ. Young siblings of children with cancer deserve care and a personalized approach. Pediatr Blood Cancer. 2008;50(3):708–710.

[4] Van Dongen-Melman JE, De Groot A, Hahlen K, Verhulst FC. Siblings of childhood cancer survivors: how does this "forgotten" group of children adjust after cessation of successful cancer treatment? Eur J Cancer. 1995 Dec;31A(13–14):2277–2283.

[5] Harding R. Children with cancer: the needs of siblings. Prof Nurse 1996;11:588–590.

[6] Carpenter PJ, Sahler OJ, Davis MS. Use of a camp setting to provide medical information to siblings of pediatric cancer patients. J Cancer Educ. 1990;5(1):21–26.

[7] Spinetta JJ, Jankovic M, Eden T, Green D, Martins AG, Wandzura C, et al. Guidelines for assistance to siblings of children with cancer: report of the SIOP Working Committee on psychosocial issues in pediatric oncology. Med Pediatr Oncol. 1999 Oct;33(4):395–398.

[8] Cullen J. Because statistics don't tell the whole story: a call for comprehensive care for children with cancer. CA Cancer J Clin. 2014 Mar–Apr;64(2):79–82.

[9] D'Urso A, Mastroyannopoulou K, Kirby A. Experiences of posttraumatic growth in siblings of children with cancer. Clin Child Psychol Psychiatry. 2016 Aug 4. 1–17.

[10] Bultz, BD, Carlson, LE. Emotional distress: the six vital sign in cancer care. J Clinical Oncol. (2005);23:6440–6441.

[11] Zabora J, Brintzenhofeszoc K, Curbow B. The prevalence of psychological distress by cancer site. Psychooncology. 2001;10:19–28

[12] Carlson LE, Angen M, Cullum J, et al. High levels of untreated distress and fatigue in cancer patients. Br J Cancer. 2004;90:2297–2304.

[13] Carlson LE, Bultz BD: Cancer distress screening: needs, methods and models. J Psychosom Res. 2003;55:403–409

[14] Lau S, Lu X, Balsamo L, Devidas M, Winick N, Hunger SP, et al. Family life events in the first year of acute lymphoblastic leukemia therapy: a children's oncology group report. Pediatr Blood Cancer. 2014 Dec;61(12):2277–2284.

[15] Tasker SL, Stonebridge GG. Siblings, You Matter: Exploring the Needs of Adolescent Siblings of Children and Youth With Cancer. J Pediatr Nurs. 2016 Nov - Dec;31(6):712-22.

[16] Prchal A, Graf A, Bergstraesser E, Landolt MA. A two-session psychological intervention for siblings of pediatric cancer patients: a randomized controlled pilot trial. Child Adolesc Psychiatr Ment Health. 2012;6:3. doi:10.1186/1753-2000-6-3.

[17] Chesler M, Allswede J, Barbairn O. Voices from the margin of the family: siblings of children with cancer. J Psychosoc Oncol. 1991; 9:19–41.

[18] Sahler O, Roghmann K, Carptenter PJ, et al. Sibling adaptation to childhood cancer collaborative study: prevalence of sibling's distress and definition of adaptation levels. J Dev Behav Pediatr. 1994;15:353–366.

[19] Barbarin O, Sahler O, Carpenter P, et al. Sibling adaptation to childhood cancer collaborative study: parental views of pre- and post-diagnosis adjustment of siblings of children with cancer. J Psychosoc Oncol. 1995;13:1–20.

[20] Harvermans T, Eiser C. Siblings of a child with cancer. Child Care Health Dev. 1994;20: 309–322.

[21] Koocher GP, O'Malley JE, editors. The Damocles syndrome: psychological consequences of surviving childhood cancer. 1981 New York: McGraw Hill.

[22] Kinrade LC. Preventive group program with siblings of oncology patients. Child Health Care. 1985;142:110–113.

[23] Hodges LJ, Humphris GM, Macfarlane G. A meta-analytic investigation of the relationship between the psychological distress of cancer patients and their carers. Soc Sci Med. 2005 Jan;60(1):1–12.

[24] Schulte F, Wurz A, Reynolds K, Strother D, Dewey D. Quality of life in survivors of pediatric cancer and their siblings: the consensus between parent-proxy and self-reports. Pediatr Blood Cancer. 2016 Apr;63(4):677–683.

[25] Spinetta JJ, Deasy-Spinetta P. Living with childhood cancer. 1981 St. Louis: Mosby.

[26] Houtzager BA, Grootenhuis MA, Caron HN, et al. Quality of life and psychological adaptation in siblings of pediatric cancer patients, 2 years after diagnosis. Psychooncology. 2003;13:499–511.

[27] Guggemos A, Juen F, Engelmann L, Diesselhorst V, Henze G, Di Gallo A. Siblings of children with cancer—the price they pay to function. Support Care Cancer. 2015 Jul;23(7):1837–1839.

[28] Woodgate RL. Siblings' experiences with childhood cancer: a different way of being in the family. Cancer Nurs. 2006 Sep–Oct;29(5):406–414.

[29] Yang HC, Mu PF, Sheng CC, Chen YW, Hung GY. A systematic review of the experiences of siblings of children with cancer. Cancer Nurs. 2016 May–Jun;39(3):E12–E21.

[30] Sidhu R, Passmore A, Baker D. An investigation into parent perceptions of the needs of siblings of children with cancer. J Pediatr Oncol Nurs. 2005;22(5):276–287.

[31] Prchal A, Landolt MA. How siblings of pediatric cancer patients experience the first time after diagnosis: a qualitative study. Cancer Nurs. 2012 Mar–Apr;35(2):133–140.

[32] Bhatia S, Robison LL, Oberlin O, Greenberg M, Bunin G, Fossati-Bellani F, et al. Breast cancer and other second neoplasms after childhood Hodgkin's disease. N Engl J Med. 1996 Mar 21;334(12):745–751.

[33] Given BA, Sherwood P, Given CW. Support for caregivers of cancer patients: transition after active treatment. Cancer Epidemiol Biomarkers Prev. 2011 Oct;20(10):2015–2021.

[34] Alderfer MA, Long KA, Lown EA, Marsland AL, Ostrowski NL, Hock JM, et al. Psychosocial adjustment of siblings of children with cancer: a systematic review. Psychooncology. 2010 Aug;19(8):789–805.

[35] Alderfer MA, Labay LE, Kazak AE. Brief report: does posttraumatic stress apply to siblings of childhood cancer survivors?. J Pediatr Psychol. 2003 Jun;28(4):281–286.

[36] Dolgin MJ, Blumensohn R, Mulhern RK, Orbach J, Sahler OJ, Roghmann KJ, et al. Sibling adaptation to childhood cancer collaborative study. J Psychosoc Oncol. 1997 Aug 15;15(1):1–14.

[37] Kamibeppu K, Sato I, Honda M, Ozono S, Sakamoto N, Iwai T, et al. Mental health among young adult survivors of childhood cancer and their siblings including posttraumatic growth. J Cancer Surviv. 2010 Dec;4(4):303–312.

[38] Tedeschi RG, Calhoun LG. The posttraumatic growth inventory: measuring the positive legacy of trauma. J Trauma Stress. 1996 Jul;9(3):455–471.

[39] Turner-Sack AM, Menna R, Setchell SR, Maan C, Cataudella D. Psychological functioning, post-traumatic growth, and coping in parents and siblings of adolescent cancer survivors. Oncol Nurs Forum. 2016 Jan;43(1):48–56.

[40] Duran B Posttraumatic growth as experienced by childhood cancer survivors and their families: a narrative synthesis of qualitative and quantitative research. J Pediatr Oncol Nurs. 2013 Jul–Aug;30(4):179–197.

[41] Howlader N, Noone AM, Krapcho M, et al. (eds). SEER Cancer Statistics Review, 1975–2011. April 2014 Bethesda, MD: National Cancer Institute, http://seer.cancer.gov/csr/1975_2011/, based on November 2013 SEER data submission, posted to the SEER web site.

[42] Lovgren M, Jalmsell L, Eilegard Wallin A, Steineck G, Kreicbergs U. Siblings' experiences of their brother's or sister's cancer death: a nationwide follow-up 2–9 years later. Psychooncology. 2016 Apr;25(4):435–440.

[43] Eilegård A, Steineck G, Nyberg T, Kreicbergs U. Psychological health in siblings who lost a brother or sister to cancer 2–9 years earlier. Psychooncology. 2013;22(3): 683–691.

[44] Rosenberg AR, Postier A, Osenga K, Kreicbergs U, Neville B, Dussel V, et al. Long-term psychosocial outcomes among bereaved siblings of children with cancer. J Pain Symptom Manage. 2015 Jan;49(1):55–65.

[45] Sveen J, Eilegard A, Steineck G, Kreicbergs U. They still grieve-a nationwide follow-up of young adults 2–9 years after losing a sibling to cancer. Psychooncology. 2014 Jun;23(6):658–664.

[46] van der Geest IM, Darlington AS, Streng IC, Michiels EM, Pieters R, van den Heuvel-Eibrink MM. Parents' experiences of pediatric palliative care and the impact on long-term parental grief. J Pain Symptom Manage. 2014 Jun;47(6):1043–1053.

[47] Di Battista A, Hancock K, Cataudella D, et al. Healthcare providers' perceptions of the utility of psychosocial screening tools in childhood cancer: a pilot study. Oncol Nurs Forum. 2015;42(4):391–397.

[48] National Institute for Health and Clinical Excellence. Improving outcomes in children and young people with cancer: Manual update. (2005) London, England: Author.

[49] Hewitt ME, Weiner SL, Simone JV. Childhood cancer survivorship: improving care and quality of life. Washington, DC: National Academies Press; 2003.

[50] Barrera M, Rokeach A, Yogalingam P, Hancock K, Johnston DL, Cataudella D, et al. Healthcare professionals' knowledge of family psychosocial problems in pediatric cancer: a pilot study. Cancer Nurs. 2016 Jul–Aug;39(4):263–271.

[51] Yogalingam P, Hancock K, Alam R, et al. The development of the psychosocial care checklist: health care practitioners' knowledge of a family's psychosocial problems. Poster presented at the Pediatric Oncology Group of Ontario Symposium; 2012; Toronto, ON.

[52] Potts S, Farrell M, O'Toole J. Treasure weekend: supporting bereaved siblings. Palliat Med. 1999;13:51–56.

[53] Lovgren M, Bylund-Grenklo T, Jalmsell L, Wallin AE, Kreicbergs U. Bereaved siblings' advice to health care professionals working with children with cancer and their families. J Pediatr Oncol Nurs. 2016 Jul;33(4):297–305.

[54] Nolbirs MJ, Nilsson S. Sibling supporters' experiences of giving support to Siblings who have a brother or a sister with cancer. J Pediatr Oncol Nurs. 2016 May;19. 1–7.

[55] Humphrey LM, Hill DL, Carroll KW, Rourke M, Kang TI, Feudtner C. Psychological well-being and family environment of siblings of children with life threatening i. J Palliat Med. 2015 Nov;18(11):981–984.

[56] Lichtenthal WG, Sweeney CR, Roberts KE, Corner GW, Donovan LA, Prigerson HG, et al. Bereavement follow-up after the death of a child as a standard of care in pediatric oncology. Pediatr Blood Cancer 2015 Dec;62 Suppl 5:S834–S869.

[57] Jones BL, Contro N, Koch KD. The duty of the physician to care for the family in pediatric palliative care: Context, communication, and caring. Pediatrics. 2014;133:S8–S15.

[58] Gerhardt CA, Lehmann V, Long KA, Alderfer MA. Supporting siblings as a standard of care in pediatric oncology. Pediatr Blood Cancer. 2015 Dec;62 Suppl 5:S750–S804.

[59] Schofield P, Carey M, Bonevski B, Sanson-Fisher R. Barriers to the provision of evidence-based psychosocial care in oncology. Psychooncology. 2006 Oct;15(10):863–872.

[60] Selove R, Kroll T, Coppes M, Cheng Y. Psychosocial services in the first 30 days after diagnosis: results of a web-based survey of children's oncology group (COG) member institutions. Pediatr Blood Cancer. 2012;58:435–440.

[61] Arceci, R. Comprehensive pediatric hematology/oncology programs: standard requirements for children and adolescents with cancer and blood disorders. 1996 Francis, R, editor. American Society of Pediatric Hematology and Oncology.

[62] Thaxter G, Stevens M, Craft A, et al. [Accessed January, 2013];Standards of care and training 2002 document. 2002 International Society of Paediatric Oncology. Available at: http://www.siop-online.org/page/standards-care-and-training-2002-document.

[63] Institute of Medicine (US) Committee on Psychosocial Services to Cancer Patients/Families in a Community Setting; Adler NE, Page AEK, editors. Cancer care for the whole patient: meeting psychosocial health needs. 2008 Washington (DC): National Academies Press (US). Available from: https://www.ncbi.nlm.nih.gov/books/NBK4015/ doi: 10.17226/11993

[64] Canadian Association of Psychosocial Oncology (CAPO) Standards of psychosocial health services for persons with cancer and their families. 2010 Toronto, ON: CAPO. [Available online at: http://www.capo.ca/CAPOstandards.pdf; cited August 18, 2011]

[65] Kowalczyk JR, Samardakiewicz M, Fitzgerald E, Essiaf S, Ladenstein R, Vassal G, et al. Towards reducing inequalities: European standards of care for children with cancer. Eur J Cancer. 2014 Feb;50(3):481–485.

[66] Kusch M, Labouvie H, Ladisch V, Fleischhack G, Bode U. Structuring psychosocial care in pediatric oncology. Patient Educ Couns. 2000 Jun;40(3):231–245.

[67] Coccia PF, Altman J, Bhatia S, Borinstein SC, Flynn J, George S, et al. Adolescent and young adult oncology. Clinical practice guidelines in oncology. J Natl Compr Canc Netw. 2012 Sep;10(9):1112–1150.

[68] Edwards MJ. Access to quality cancer care: consensus statement of the American Federation of Clinical Oncologic Societies. Ann Surg Oncol. 1998 Oct–Nov;5(7):657–659.

[69] Clarke, S; Mitchell, W; Sloper, P Social policy research unit. 2004 York: University of York. Care and Support Needs of Children and Young People with Cancer and Leukaemia and Their Families.

[70] Zebrack B, Mathews-Bradshaw B, Siegel S, LIVESTRONG Young Adult Alliance. Quality cancer care for adolescents and young adults: a position statement. J Clin Oncol. 2010 Nov 10;28(32):4862–4867.

[71] Centers for Disease Control and Prevention. Health-related quality of life. 2012. www.cdc.gov/hrqol/. Accessed July 18, 2015.

[72] Patel SK, Mullins W, Turk A, Dekel N, Kinjo C, Sato JK. Distress screening, rater agreement, and services in pediatric oncology. Psychooncology. 2011 Dec;20(12):1324–1333.

[73] Kazak AE, Prusak A, McSherry M, et al. The psychosocial assessment tool (PAT): development of a brief screening instrument for identifying high risk families in pediatric oncology. Fam Syst Health. 2001;19:303–317.

[74] Pai AL, Patiño-Fernández AM, McSherry M, et al. The psychosocial assessment tool (PAT2.0): psychometric properties of a screener for psychosocial distress in families of children newly diagnosed with cancer. J Pediatr Psychol. 2008;33(1):50–62.

Chapter 5

Evaluation and Long-Term Outcomes of Cardiac Toxicity in Paediatric Cancer Patients

Jake A. Kleinmahon and Bruce F. Landeck, II

Additional information is available at the end of the chapter

http://dx.doi.org/10.5772/67043

Abstract

Paediatric cancer survival rates have increased dramatically in the last 20 years. With decreased mortality comes increased long-term morbidity. Cardiovascular disease is the leading cause of secondary morbidity and mortality of childhood cancer survivors. The most common chemotherapeutic agents in treatment regimens are implicated in chemotherapy-induced cardiomyopathy. The clinical presentation is rarely uniform and may manifest in symptoms besides chest pain, shortness of breath or decreased exercise tolerance. In addition to symptomatic patients, asymptomatic patients are especially important to screen as the effects of cardiac toxicity are reversible if caught early. There are new techniques more sensitive than traditional 2D echocardiography ejection fraction that may lead to earlier detection of cardiac dysfunction. Treatment methods have changed little in the recent past with the exception of miniaturization of support devices allowing for cardiac recovery or bridge to cardiac transplant.

Keywords: cardiomyopathy, cardio-oncology, heart failure, cardiotoxicity, anthracyclines

1. Introduction

Cardiovascular compromise is the leading cause of morbidity and mortality of childhood cancer survivors [1]. As paediatric cancer treatment improves and survival increases, there is a significant amount of that population with resultant secondary morbidities who need to be monitored. Paediatric cancer survivors have been found to have an eight-time greater risk of dying from a cardiovascular event compared to their peers [2]. Routine monitoring is paramount because progressive cardiac dysfunction in children may not be present in typical fashion [3]. Children may also be too young to effectively communicate what they are feeling, requiring the provider to obtain a specific history from the caretaker, a detailed physical exam and often adjunct imaging and laboratory studies. When cardiac dysfunction is found early, working with the oncology team to limit further cardiotoxic medications, if possible, as well as implementing heart failure management strategies may lead to full cardiac recovery.

2. Clinical presentation and initial assessment

Depending on the chemotherapeutic agent used, heart failure can present in 0.5–28% of patients [2], and a larger percentage can have other cardiac-related dysfunctions. The typical presentation of heart failure is dyspnoea, oedema and chest pain [4]. However, more than half of patients who present to an emergency department for cardiomyopathies have a primary complaint of gastrointestinal symptoms such as abdominal pain, decreased appetite, nausea or vomiting. Symptoms can be often vague, and a high index of suspicion is needed to prompt further evaluation. In babies, the history should include questions such as changes in feeding patterns, decreased tolerance of feeds, tiring or sweating with feeds and poor weight gain. In older children, the history should include questions about keeping up with peers, changes in weight (either increased or decreased), puffiness, nausea or vomiting, decreased appetite, overall level of energy and if they're needing more pillows to sleep on at night. Asymptomatic patients may also have small decreases in cardiac function that can be clinically important.

The physical exam should include vital signs such as heart rate, blood pressure, pulse oximetry, respiratory rate, weight and height. A thorough cardiac exam includes palpation of the chest wall for chest wall abnormalities as well as feeling for a point of maximal impulse. When auscultating it is important to assess for murmurs, an abnormally split S2, an S3 or S4, a P2, as well as a rub or distant heart sounds. Jugular venous distension should be noted as well as any carotid bruits. The extremities should be examined for pulses, oedema, capillary refill or nodules. The nail beds should be examined looking for splinter haemorrhages as a sign of endocarditis. The abdomen should be palpated for liver and spleen size if able.

These patients have accelerated coronary artery disease [5] that can have a varying presentation from being asymptomatic to acute coronary syndrome and myocardial infarction. Hypertension manifests in this patient population secondary to reduced nitric oxide production, and screening blood pressures should be obtained during clinic visits [6]. Longstanding hypertension can lead to left ventricular hypertrophy and ultimately dysfunction. Paediatric cancer survivors are also at risk for increased thromboembolic events and may present with tachycardia, chest pain, shortness of breath and symptoms, which could be due to pulmonary embolism. Patients with unilateral leg pain should be worked up for deep vein thromboses.

3. Common cardiotoxic agents

Many conventional forms of chemotherapy are aimed at causing cancer cell injury and death; however, they can also induce myocardial cell damage. This injury from agents such as anthracyclines, antimetabolites and cyclophosphamide can lead to acute or chronic left ventricular dysfunction [2]. Right ventricular dysfunction is rare, but some drugs such as anthracyclines, cyclophosphamide and 5-fluouracil can cause right ventricular systolic and diastolic function [7]. It is important to be aware of the offending agents in order to minimize exposure, if clinically possible, in a failing heart. Left ventricular dysfunction from anthracycline exposure has been well studied and is dose dependent. Thus, it is important to have a clear record of the lifetime dosage a patient receives of chemotherapeutic agents. **Table 1** lists the most common cardiotoxic agents and their toxic dose ranges.

Every patient is different, which is why routine screening of cardiac dysfunction is recommended even below the toxic level range as well as with drugs not typically associated with cardiac dysfunction. Radiation can also be cardiotoxic leading to myocardial oedema, fibrosis and necrosis, and total radiation dose as well as the area radiated should be recorded.

Drug	Toxic dose range	Cardiac toxicity	Frequency
Doxorubicin	>450 mg/m^2	LV dysfunction	>5% [6]
Epirubicin	>900 mg/m^2	LV dysfunction	>5% [6]
Idarubicin	150–290 mg/m^2	LV dysfunction, heart failure	5–18% [8]
Docetaxel		Arrhythmia, heart failure	5% [9]
Cyclophosphamide	>100–120 mg/kg	LV dysfunction	2–10% [9]
Ifosfamide	>10 mg/m^2	Arrhythmias	Unknown
Capecitabine	Conventional dose	Cardiac ischemia	1–18% [10]
Fluorouracil	Conventional dose	Arrhythmias, myocardial ischemia	1–18% [10]
Arsenic trioxide	Conventional dose	QTc prolongation	>5% [6]
Cisplatin		Diastolic dysfunction, myocardial ischemia, hypertension [11]	>6% (major cardiac event)

Table 1. Common cardiotoxic chemotherapeutic agents and their cardiotoxicity.

4. Screening

4.1. Electrocardiography

A baseline electrocardiogram (ECG) should be obtained on all patients before undergoing chemotherapy. ECGs are relatively inexpensive, quick and noninvasive screening tests that give information about chamber sizes, depolarization abnormalities, rhythm disturbances and conduction abnormalities. Some of the chemotherapeutic agents or supportive medications prolong QT intervals so it is important to manually calculate a QTc before initiating therapy as well as while on QT-prolonging medications. ECGs can be repeated during imaging follow-up or with any concerning symptoms. Twenty-four hour Holter monitors should be ordered as clinically indicated.

4.2. Echocardiography

Echocardiography is the most widely used imaging modality for screening cardiac dysfunction and is an important noninvasive manner to follow up cardiac function over time. The advantages of echocardiography are that it is widely available in paediatric cardiology clinics, can usually be performed without sedation and is noninvasive, and a targeted function exam can be performed relatively quickly in the inpatient and outpatient setting. It is recommended that all patients have a complete paediatric echocardiogram before the initiation of chemotherapy. All structures of the heart should be visualized including coronary arteries, the pulmonary veins and the aortic arch during the first echocardiogram. If all structures are seen adequately during the first echocardiogram, subsequent echocardiograms can be targeted function exams. The cardiac valves should be visualized on all exams as these patients have an increased risk of endocarditis, nonbacterial thrombotic endocarditis as well as radiation-induced heart disease affecting valves [7]. Transthoracic echocardiography is acceptable for looking for endocarditis if there are clear windows to the heart valves; otherwise depending on the index of suspicion, transoesophageal echocardiography is indicated as the gold standard.

Surveillance echocardiograms, or equivalent cardiac imaging, should be performed anywhere from yearly to every 5 years depending on doxorubicin isotoxic equivalent dosing, age and radiation for asymptomatic children with stable function [12]. It is recommended that any decrease in serial function should be assessed yearly. Also, patients with clinical changes should be assessed more frequently.

Historically, left ventricular ejection fraction (EF) has been used to quantitate cardiac function over time. While EF is an adequate gross marker of cardiac function, it may not be sensitive enough to detect early cardiac dysfunction [13–15]. Zito et al. demonstrated that there is enough variability in EF measurements that it is not sensitive to detect a decrease in EF less than 10% [7]. If one is using EF as their main determinant of cardiac function, they may miss patients who have a significant decrease in cardiac function that may alter the course of therapy.

Some centres rely on indices of cardiac function other than EF. Strain and strain rate have been found to detect cardiac dysfunction earlier than a decrease in LV systolic function [16]. Strain is a measure of myocardial deformation or the fractional change in the length of a myocardial segment. Strain can be measured by tissue Doppler imaging (TDI) as well as speckle-tracking echocardiography (STE). Each of these methods requires adequate 2D echocardiographic imaging windows in order to process the image. TDI is angle dependent, requiring the plane of the ultrasound to be in line with the tissue being interrogated. One benefit of STE is that it is not angle dependent. Speckle tracking can determine peak systolic global longitudinal strain (GLS), which is becoming a commonly accepted method for evaluating myocardial function [17]. **Figures 1** and **2** demonstrate examples of normal vs abnormal global and regional strain, respectively. This method is quite useful for early detection of cardiotoxicity. It is likely that all of these indices used in conjunction with one another will provide the best insight to the cardiac status of the patient.

Diastolic function must also be evaluated during an echocardiographic evaluation of a paediatric cancer patient. Diastolic dysfunction may proceed to systolic deterioration and can indicate a need for closer follow-up as it has been reported that it can be a predictor of subsequent deterioration [18]. Diastolic dysfunction can be detected with a decrease in early to late ventricular filling velocities (E/A ratio), an increased E/e′ ratio, enlargement of the atria and an increase in isovolumic relaxation time. TDI-derived peak early and late diastolic myocardial velocities of the right ventricular free wall, left ventricular lateral wall and septum are decreased in patients with myocardial dysfunction when compared with controls [19].

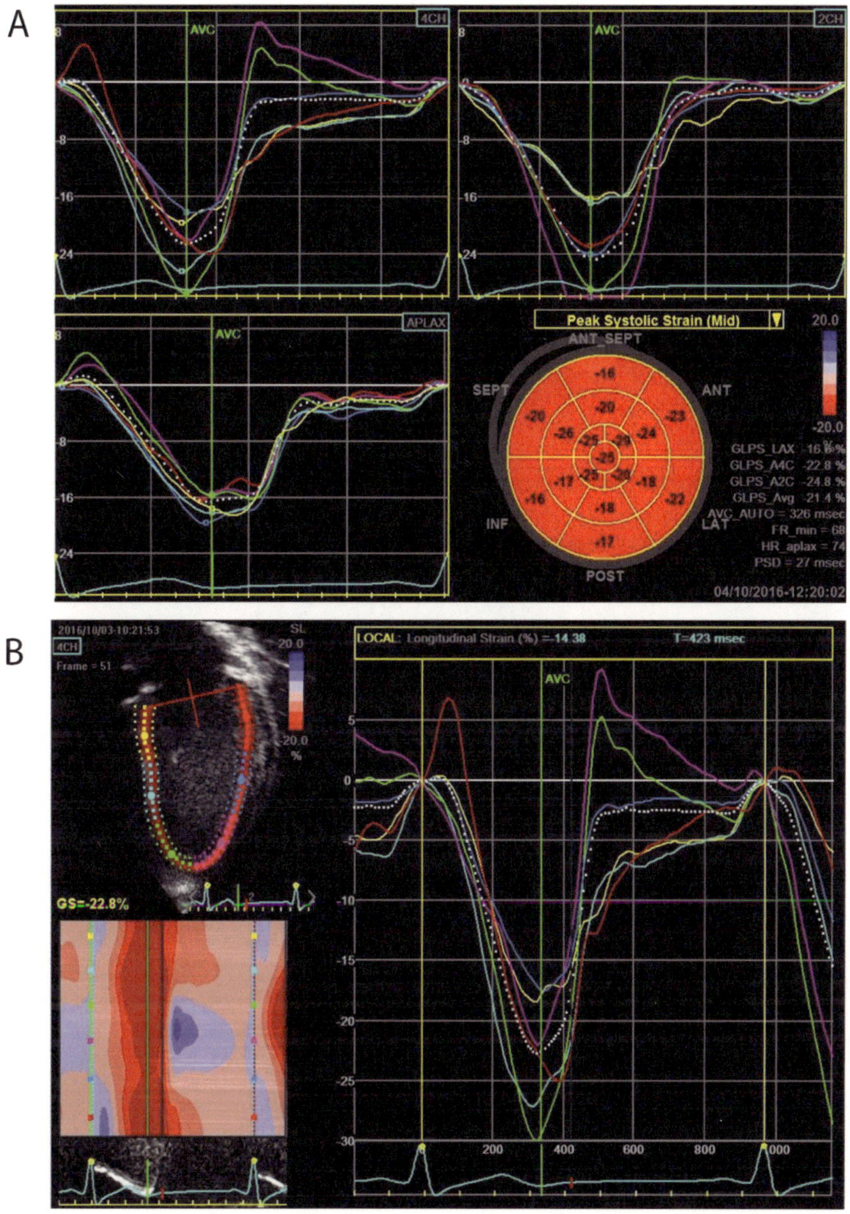

Figure 1. (A) Longitudinal strain analysis of the left ventricle, with both regional and global longitudinal strain reported. The six segment strain curves from the apical 4-chamber, apical 2-chamber and apical long axis are shown, as well as a "bullseye" view overlaying the longitudinal strain for each segment. (B) Segmental strain for the apical 4-chamber view, including contours of the left ventricle. Global longitudinal strain of the entire 4-chamber slice is normal at −22.8%.

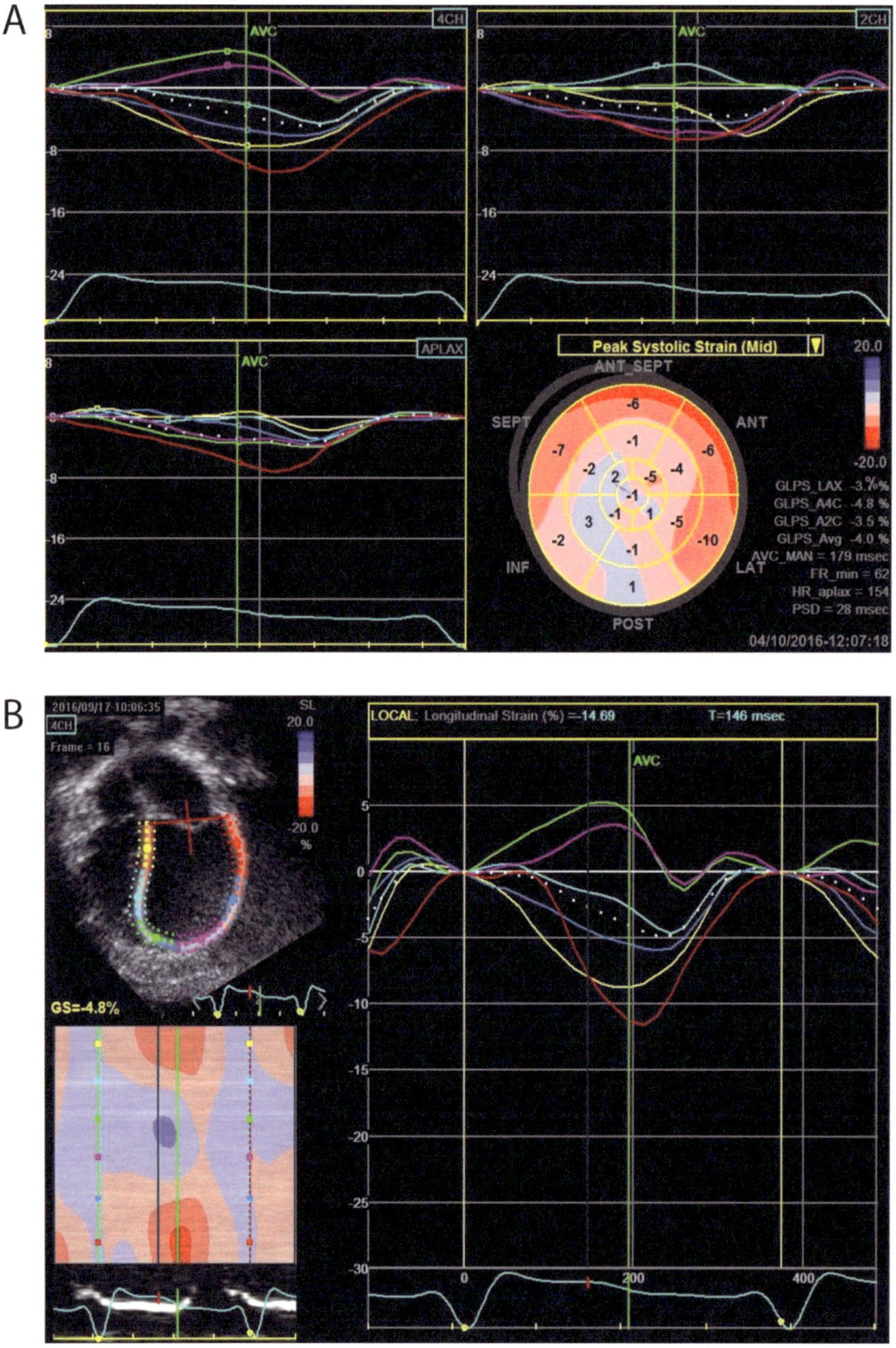

Figure 2. (A) Abnormally diminished regional and global longitudinal strain in a patient who has anthracycline-induced cardiomyopathy. Note the decreased regional strain values in nearly every segment, including positive strain (stretch of the muscle) during systole, indicating dyssynchrony. (B) Abnormally diminished global longitudinal strain of the entire 4-chamber slice at −4.8%. Note the strain waveforms above baseline which represent segments stretching during systole instead of contracting (indicative of dyssynchrony).

http://dx.doi.org/10.5772/67043

Three-dimensional echocardiography is being increasingly used as a more accurate measurement of left ventricular systolic function. Where, as previously described, 2D EF may be an inadequate measurement of systolic function, 3D echocardiography is a more sensitive method to detect decreased LV contractility than fractional shortening by M-mode or EF by 2D [20]. **Figure 3** shows an example of how 3D echocardiography is used clinically in patients receiving anthracyclines. If the patient has poor acoustic windows, however, 3D measurements will be unsatisfactory as these measurements rely on clear 2D acquisition. Besides EF, 3D speckle-tracking echocardiography is an emerging technique [4]. A 3D evaluation avoids the geometric assumptions of 2D imaging and shows good correlation of decreased myocardial contractility compared to MRI findings. At this time, 3D STE is largely experimental and not widely available in most echo laboratories.

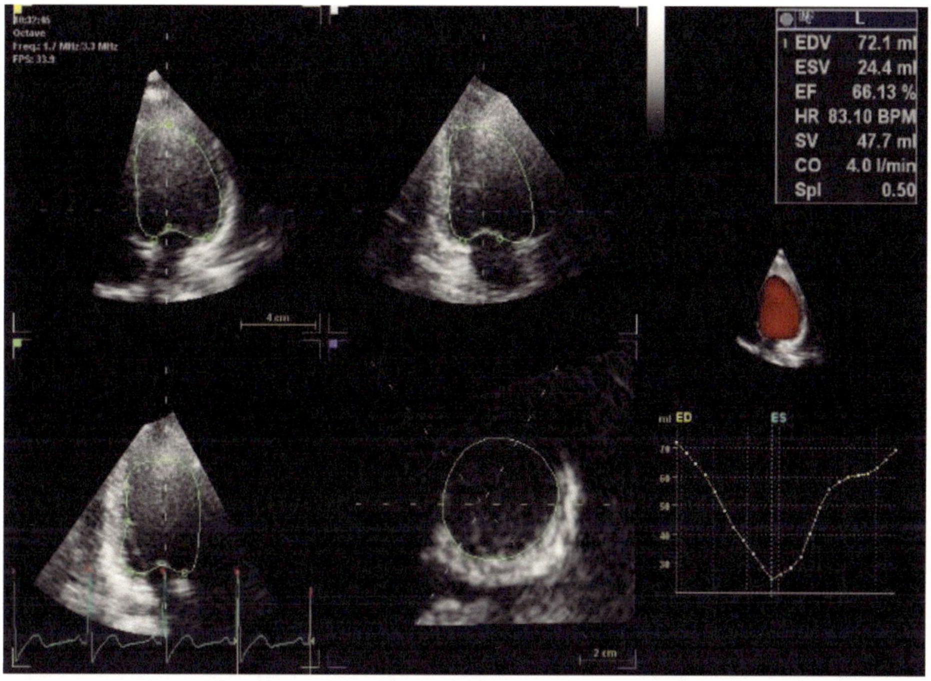

Figure 3. A three-dimensional reconstruction of the left ventricle in a patient receiving anthracyclines. Care is taken to show accurate contouring of the endocardial border in multiple imaging planes. Output includes end-diastolic volume, end-systolic volume and ejection fraction.

4.3. Cardiac magnetic resonance imaging

Cardiac magnetic resonance imaging (CMRI) is increasingly playing a larger role in the imaging of paediatric cancer survivors. It allows for tissue characterization, identification of areas of fibrosis or oedema as well as a more precise and reproducible measurement of cardiac function than echocardiography. There is no need in CMRI for the geometrical assumptions to inherent in 2D echo, which can lead to imprecise echocardiographic measurements, and there is no need for optimal acoustic windows [21]. In paediatric cancer patients, minimal decreases in systolic function may lead to a change in management; thus, a sensitive method such as CMRI is useful for monitoring.

Chemotherapy, as expected, can produce myocardial changes such as tissue fibrosis, oedema and even necrosis. Other imaging modalities are not as sensitive as CMRI in detecting these changes, and CMRI may help in determining a nidus for an arrhythmia or differentiating potentially reversible vs. irreversible causes of myocardial depression. T2-weighted sequences are useful for determining oedema as these areas reveal a hyperintense signal. There is evidence that myocardial oedema is related to subsequent decreased RV function. T2 mapping can also be used to follow the course of a patient over time. The clinical benefit of this is being investigated and with time it is likely that there will be a more useful correlation with clinical outcomes [21]. Late gadolinium enhancement is useful in detecting areas of fibrosis or ischemia and can help determine prognosis in cardiomyopathies [22]. **Figure 4** shows an example of how CMRI can be used to detect scar and fibrosis by late gadolinium enhancement. This technique uses a T1 inversion sequence about 10 minutes after injection of a gadolinium-based contrast. CMRI can also quantify myocardial perfusion, helpful for the diagnosis of coronary artery disease [23].

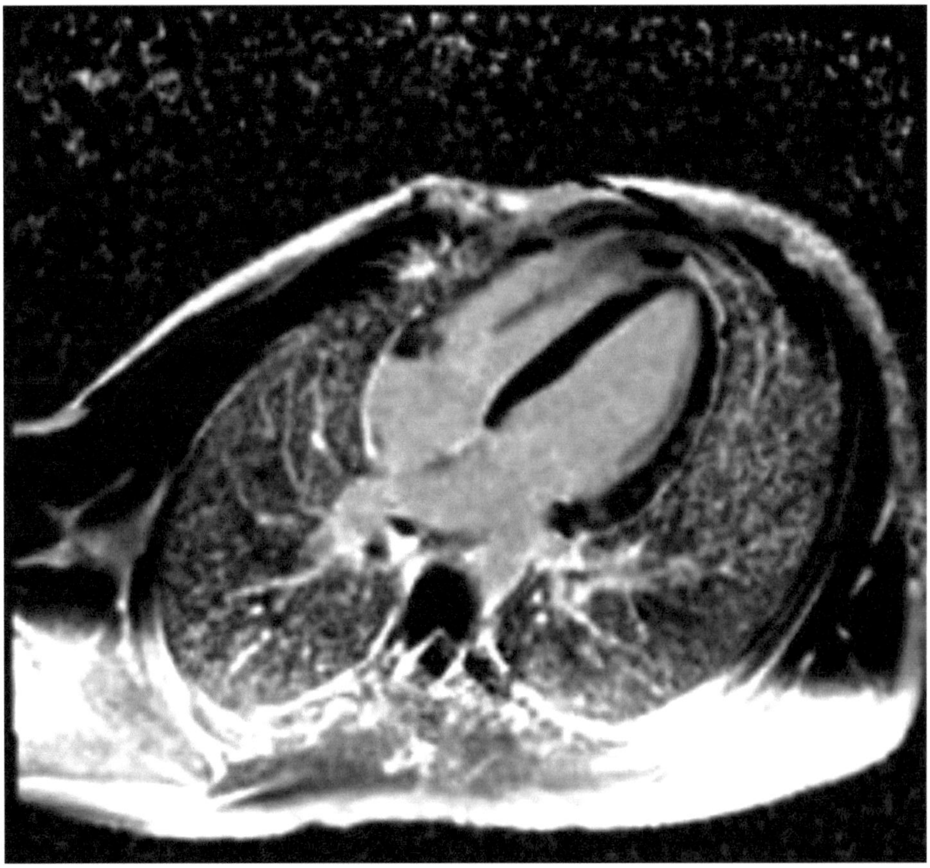

Figure 4. Cardiac MRI demonstrating scar and fibrosis using a late gadolinium enhancement technique.

While 3D echocardiography is emerging, CMRI has a higher sensitivity of detecting a left ventricular ejection fraction <50% [24]. CMRI is also useful in characterization of the right

http://dx.doi.org/10.5772/67043

ventricle because of its irregular shape that is not amenable to geometrical formulas. Although right ventricular dysfunction is not as common as left ventricular dysfunction in paediatric heart transplant survivors, its consequences can be just as severe.

CMRI can have its downside, especially in children, as it requires the patient to lie still, which may be difficult for young children. Anaesthesia is often necessary for an optimal exam of a child. Also, because most CMRI images require ECG gating CMRI and be difficult or impossible in the setting of arrhythmias. Metallic implants are often contraindicated with CMRI, or if placed in the thorax, they may produce significant artefact, which obscures images.

5. Biomarkers

Biomarkers can be used in conjunction with history, physical examination and imaging modalities to gather information on a patient's clinical status. Unfortunately, there is no single biomarker that can predict the cardiac prognosis of a patient.

Cardiac troponins are a widely used biomarker in the field of cardiology and have been found to be useful in evaluating anthracycline-induced cardiomyopathies [25]. Troponin I and troponin T are both sensitive and specific to cardiac damage. The troponin complex is on the thin filament of the contraction mechanism and is important in excitation-contraction coupling in the heart [26]. Cardiac troponin I increases with anthracycline exposure and appears to be dose related. Increased cardiac troponin T levels in the first 90 days of therapy have been shown to correlate with cardiotoxicity at 4 years of follow-up [25].

B-Natriuretic peptide (BNP) and NT-pro-B-natriuretic peptide (proBNP) are closely related cardiac biomarkers that can aid clinical management of heart failure. Impaired ventricular function leads to greater wall stress, which triggers the synthesis of pre-pro-B-type natriuretic; this is then broken down to proBNP and then cleaved to BNP. The purpose of these peptides is to protect the body from volume overload. BNP and proBNP are related but cannot be used interchangeably as their reference values are different. Also, the half-life of BNP is about 20 min where proBNP is about 1–2 h. The result of the release of BNP is smooth muscle and myocardial relaxation and diuresis and natriuresis [27]. BNP is elevated in children with anthracycline-induced clinical or subclinical heart failure and can be used along with imaging to trend the degree of heart failure [28].

Highly sensitive C-reactive protein (hsCRP) has been shown to predict cardiac events in adults; however, this was not found to be true in the paediatric population with heart failure, so it is not recommended for routine monitoring [29].

6. Management of cardiomyopathy

The best way to manage heart failure secondary to chemotherapy is to have a robust monitoring programme to prevent its occurrence in the first place. Aggressive medical management should begin in the asymptomatic patient once early signs of ventricular dysfunction are detected [30]. Cardiotoxic medications should be avoided or minimized if possible to attempt to halt further progression.

There are few large multicentre studies in the paediatric literature to guide heart failure management so we extrapolate data from adults and apply many of the same principles to paediatric heart failure. The common classes of drugs to treat chemotherapy-induced cardiomyopathy include beta-blockers and angiotensin-converting enzyme inhibitors (ACEis).

6.1. Beta-blockers

Beta-blockers are the most effective when used shortly after anthracycline-induced cardiac injury [6]. Beta-blockers have been found to improve cardiac recovery when used as monotherapy or in combination with ACEi. Beta-blockers blunt heart rate responses so immunocompromised patients on beta-blockers should be monitored closely as their compensatory heart rate response may be blunted in times of stress. Adult trials of metoprolol and bisoprolol found that those drugs improve symptoms and survival in mild-to-moderate heart failure [31, 32]. Beta-blockers can be titrated based on heart rate response, and effective doses vary depending on the patient. The mechanism of beta-blockers in heart failure management is not completely clear but is thought to have reversed remodelling effects secondary to myocyte damage from prolonged adrenergic activation.

6.2. Angiotensin-converting enzyme inhibitors

ACEis are also commonly used in the management of heart failure secondary to chemotherapeutic cardiotoxicity. ACEis have the ability to decrease cardiac work by decreasing preload, afterload and wall stress [33]. They are also felt to improve cardiac remodelling. They should be used with caution in patients with renal insufficiency or concurrent treatment with nephrotoxic medications. Renal function should be monitored regularly, especially when titrating dose. There are several adult studies that showed benefit with ACEi in regard to mortality. One in particular suggests that a combination of enalapril and carvedilol (a beta-blocker) may increase left ventricular EF when started at the earliest signs of cardiac dysfunction [34]. In children, however, enalapril did not reveal an improvement in cardiac function [35].

6.3. Statins

Statins are not as widely used in the paediatric population but have antioxidative and anti-inflammatory effects and may play a role in prevention of cardiotoxicity. In adults, a retrospective case-control study revealed that patients who received statins at the time of anthracycline treatment had a lower incidence of HF at 2.5 years follow-up [36]. Statins are safe in children with the proper monitoring; however, their effects on chemotherapy-induced cardiomyopathy are unknown.

6.4. Ventricular assist devices

Ventricular assist devices (VADs) can now be considered in children with inotropic-dependent heart failure. The miniaturization of VAD is allowing for more children to be potential candidates with newer devices supporting lower body surface areas and weights. Most often, chemotherapy-induced cardiomyopathies are slow to recover function if at all so VAD can be used as a bridge to transplant or in some cases, recovery [23]. VAD can allow patients to be discharged from the hospital, while they are awaiting a heart transplant or recovery. These devices are not without risks, however. Complications such as bleeding, thromboemboli or infection are not uncommon and require close monitoring. The proximity to the hospital as well as the social support system should also be considered when deciding to implant a VAD in a patient.

6.5. Heart transplantation

The definitive treatment for heart failure not responsive to medical therapy is transplantation. Some centres consider transplantation if a patient has been cancer-free for 5 years and are not requiring ongoing cardiotoxic medications. There may be exceptions based on the clinical picture. Unfortunately, immunosuppressive medications required for heart transplants decrease the body's ability to detect and destroy cancer cells so it is not uncommon for secondary malignancies to occur. While transplantation can be life-saving, the cardiac graft has a limited lifespan so the decision to proceed with transplantation should be carefully weighed.

7. Conclusion

Cardiac dysfunctions secondary to cancer treatments are not uncommon. Unfortunately, there have been few breakthrough treatment modalities to treat childhood cancer survivors with heart failure; thus, it is important that these patients are having routine cardiac surveillance to detect cardiac dysfunction before it is severe or the patient is symptomatic. This would allow for altering the treatment plan as well as starting on supportive therapy earlier, which may be beneficial allowing for full cardiac recovery. Institutions should develop robust protocols and have close collaboration with oncologists and cardiologists to ensure that these patients are receiving optimal care.

Author details

Jake A. Kleinmahon* and Bruce F. Landeck, II

*Address all correspondence to: jake.kleinmahon@childrenscolorado.org

University of Colorado School of Medicine, Children's Hospital of Colorado, Aurora, CO, USA

References

[1] Lipshultz SE, Karnik R, Sambatakos P, Franco VI, Ross SW, Miller TL. Anthracycline-related cardiotoxicity in childhood cancer survivors. *Current Opinion in Cardiology*. 2014;29(1):103–112. doi:10.1097/HCO.0000000000000034.

[2] Yeh ETH, Bickford CL. Cardiovascular complications of cancer therapy. *Journal of the American College of Cardiology*. 2009;53(24):2231–2247. doi:10.1016/j.jacc.2009.02.050.

[3] Lenihan DJ, Hartlage G, DeCara J, et al.. Cardio-oncology training: a proposal from the International cardioncology society and Canadian cardiac oncology network for a new multidisciplinary specialty. *Journal of Cardiac Failure*. 2016;22(6):465–471. doi:10.1016/j.cardfail.2016.03.012.

[4] Vizzari G, Qamar R, Bomzer C, Carerj S, Zito C, Khandheria BK. Review article multimodality imaging in cardiooncology. *Journal of Oncology* August 2015:1–9. doi: 10.1155/2015/263950.

[5] Brassareo P. Cardiotoxicity from anthracycline and cardioprotection in paediatric cancer patients. *Journal of Cardiovascular Medicine*. 2016;17:e55–e63.

[6] Curigliano G, Cardinale D, Dent S, et al. Cardiotoxicity of anticancer treatments: epidemiology, detection, and management. *CA: A Cancer Journal for Clinicians*. 2016;66(4):309–325. doi:10.3322/caac.21341.

[7] Zito C, Longobardo L, Cadeddu C, et al. Cardiovascular imaging in the diagnosis and monitoring of cardiotoxicity. *Journal of Cardiovascular Medicine*. 2016;17:e35–e44. doi:10.2459/JCM.0000000000000374.

[8] Anderlini P, Benjamin RS, Wong FC, et al. Idarubicin cardiotoxicity: a retrospective study in acute myeloid leukemia and myelodysplasia. *Journal of Clinical Oncology*. 1995; 13(11):2827–2834.

[9] Schimmel KJM, Richel DJ, van den Brink RBA, Guchelaar HJ. Cardiotoxicity of cytotoxic drugs. *Cancer Treatment Reviews*. 2004;30(2):181–191. doi:10.1016/j.ctrv.2003.07.003.

[10] Ang C, Kornbluth M, Thirlwell MP, Rajan RD. Capecitabine-induced cardiotoxicity: case report and review of the literature. *Current Oncology*. 2010;17(1):59–63.

[11] Meinardi MT, Gietema JA, van der Graaf WT, et al. Cardiovascular morbidity in long-term survivors of metastatic testicular cancer. *Journal of Clinical Oncology*. 2000; 18(8):1725–1732.

[12] Children's Oncology Group. Long-Term Follow-Up Guidelines for Survivors of Childhood, Adolescent, and Young Adult Cancers. Vol 4. Arcadia; 2013.

[13] Moon TJ, Miyamoto SD, Younoszai AK, Landeck BF. Left ventricular strain and strain rates are decreased in children with normal fractional shortening after exposure to anthracycline chemotherapy. *Cardiology in Young*. 2013;24(05):854–865. doi:10.1017/S1047951113001182.

[14] Sawaya H, Sebag IA, Plana JC, et al.. Assessment of echocardiography and biomarkers for the extended prediction of cardiotoxicity in patients treated with anthracyclines, taxanes, and trastuzumab. *Circulation. Cardiovascular Imaging*. 2012;5(5):596–603. doi:10.1161/CIRCIMAGING.112.973321.

[15] Narayan HK, French B, Khan AM, et al.. Noninvasive measures of ventricular-arterial coupling and circumferential strain predict cancer therapeutics-related cardiac dysfunction. *JACC. Cardiovascular Imaging*. April 2016. doi:10.1016/j.jcmg.2015.11.024.

[16] Chen-Scarabelli C, McRee C, Leesar MA, Hage FG, Scarabelli TM. Comprehensive review on cardio-oncology: role of multimodality imaging. *Journal of Nuclear Cardiology*. May 2016:1–30. doi:10.1007/s12350-016-0535-y.

[17] Tei C, Ling LH, Hodge DO, Bailey KR, Oh JK, Rodeheffer RJ, Tajik AJ, Seward JB. New index of combined systolic and diastolic myocardial performance: a simple and reproducible measure of cardiac function—a study in normals and dilated cardiomyopathy. *Journal of Cardiology*. 1995;6:357–366.

[18] Stoddard MF, Seeger J, Liddell NE, Hadley TJ, Sullivan DM, Kupersmith J. Prolongation of isovolumetric relaxation time as assessed by Doppler echocardiography predicts doxorubicin-induced systolic dysfunction in humans. *Journal of the American College of Cardiology*. 1992;20(1):62–69.

[19] Yağci-Küpeli B, Varan A, Yorgun H, Kaya B, Büyükpamukçu M. Tissue Doppler and myocardial deformation imaging to detect myocardial dysfunction in pediatric cancer patients treated with high doses of anthracyclines. *Asia-Pacific Journal of Clinical Oncology*. 2012;8(4):368–374. doi:10.1111/j.1743-7563.2012.01566.x.

[20] Poutanen T. Long-term prospective follow-up study of cardiac function after cardiotoxic therapy for malignancy in children. *Journal of Clinical Oncology*. 2003;21(12):2349–2356. doi:10.1200/JCO.2003.08.050.

[21] Pepe A, Pizzino F, Gargiulo P, et al.. Cardiovascular imaging in the diagnosis and monitoring of cardiotoxicity. *Journal of Cardiovascular Medicine*. 2016;17:e45–e54. doi:10.2459/JCM.0000000000000380.

[22] Mahrholdt H, Wagner A, Judd RM, Sechtem U, Kim RJ. Delayed enhancement cardiovascular magnetic resonance assessment of non-ischaemic cardiomyopathies. *European Heart Journal*. 2005;26(15):1461–1474. doi:10.1093/eurheartj/ehi258.

[23] Wickramasinghe CD, Nguyen KL, Watson KE, Vorobiof G, Yang EH. Concepts in cardio-oncology: definitions, mechanisms, diagnosis and treatment strategies of cancer therapy-induced cardiotoxicity. *Future Oncology*. 2016;12(6):855–870. doi:10.2217/fon.15.349.

[24] Armstrong GT, Plana JC, Zhang N, et al.. Screening adult survivors of childhood cancer for cardiomyopathy: comparison of echocardiography and cardiac magnetic resonance imaging. *Journal of Clinical Oncology*. 2012;30(23):2876–2884. doi:10.1200/JCO.2011.40.3584.

[25] Henri C, Heinonen T, Tardif JC. The role of biomarkers in decreasing risk of cardiac toxicity after cancer therapy. *BIC*. May 2016:39–7. doi:10.4137/BIC.S31798.

[26] Rubini Gimenez M, Twerenbold R, Reichlin T, et al.. Direct comparison of high-sensitivity-cardiac troponin I versus T for the early diagnosis of acute myocardial infarction. *European Heart Journal*. 2014;35(34):2303–2311. doi:10.1093/eurheartj/ehu188.

[27] Allen HD, Driscoll DJ, Shaddy RE, Feltes TF. Moss & Adams' Heart Disease in Infants, Children, and Adolescents, Including the Fetus and Young Adult. Vol 2. 8th ed. Lippincott Williams & Wilkins: New South Wales; 2016:1567–1569.

[28] Aggarwal S, Pettersen MD, Bhambhani K, Gurczynski J, Thomas R, L'Ecuyer T. B-type natriuretic peptide as a marker for cardiac dysfunction in anthracycline-treated children. *Pediatric Blood & Cancer*. 2007;49(6):812–816. doi:10.1002/pbc.21100.

[29] Lipshultz SE, Miller TL, Scully RE, et al. Changes in cardiac biomarkers during doxorubicin treatment of pediatric patients with high-risk acute lymphoblastic leukemia: associations with long-term echocardiographic outcomes. *Journal of Clinical Oncology*. 2012;30(10):1042–1049. doi:10.1200/JCO.2010.30.3404.

[30] Bovelli D, Plataniotis G, Roila F, ESMO Guidelines Working Group. Cardiotoxicity of chemotherapeutic agents and radiotherapy-related heart disease: ESMO clinical practice guidelines. *Annals Oncology*. 2010;21(Suppl 5):v277–v282. doi:10.1093/annonc/mdq200.

[31] MERIT-HF Study Group, Effect of metoprolol CR/XL in chronic heart failure: Metoprolol CR/XL randomised intervention trial in-congestive heart failure (MERIT-HF). *The Lancet*. 1999;353(9169):2001–2007. doi:10.1016/S0140-6736(99)04440-2.

[32] CIBIS-II Investigators and Committees, The cardiac insufficiency bisoprolol study II (CIBIS-II): a randomised trial. *The Lancet*. 1999;353(9146):9–13. doi:10.1016/S0140-6736(98)11181-9.

[33] Cruz M, Duarte-Rodrigues J, Campelo M. Cardiotoxicity in anthracycline therapy: Prevention strategies. *Revista Portuguesa de Cardiologia (English Edition)*. June 2016:1–13. doi:10.1016/j.repce.2015.12.020.

[34] Cardinale D, Colombo A, Lamantia G, et al. Anthracycline-induced cardiomyopathy: clinical relevance and response to pharmacologic therapy. *Journal of the American College of Cardiology*. 2010;55(3):213–220. doi:10.1016/j.jacc.2009.03.095.

[35] Silber JH, Cnaan A, Clark BJ, et al. Enalapril to prevent cardiac function decline in long-term survivors of pediatric cancer exposed to anthracyclines. *Journal of Clinical Oncology*. 2004;22(5):820–828. doi:10.1200/JCO.2004.06.022.

[36] Seicean S, Seicean A, Plana JC, Budd GT, Marwick TH. Effect of statin therapy on the risk for incident heart failure in patients with breast cancer receiving anthracycline chemotherapy. *Journal of the American College of Cardiology*. 2012;60(23):2384–2390. doi:10.1016/j.jacc.2012.07.067.

Chapter 6

Long-Term Survivors of Childhood Cancer: The Late Effects of Therapy

Nupur Mittal and Paul Kent

Additional information is available at the end of the chapter

http://dx.doi.org/10.5772/67366

Abstract

The overall cure rate for pediatric malignancies is significantly improved to over 75% with an estimated 270,000 survivors of childhood cancer in the United States currently. The achievement of high cure rates for most pediatric malignancies has been accompanied by a growing population of childhood cancer survivors who are at an increased risk for a myriad of health problems resulting from their cancer or its treatment. Some cancer-related complications do not become apparent until several years following cancer treatment. As the survivors of childhood cancers age, the effects of therapy may be exacerbated by effects of aging on organ function. Late effects encompass a variety of detrimental conditions including organ dysfunction, psychosocial complications, and subsequent malignancies that may negatively impact quality of life and may predispose them to early mortality. In contrast to the multitude of publications describing treatment-related sequelae in childhood cancer survivors, relatively few provide specific recommendations for health screening and risk-reduction counseling to guide healthcare providers in monitoring this vulnerable population. In this chapter, we will summarize the evaluation and management of childhood cancer survivors who may be encountered across a wide variety of healthcare settings, salient issues influencing healthcare for childhood cancer survivors, of which guidelines currently available and limitations in current practice.

Keywords: late effects, pediatric oncology, cancer survivors, long-term follow-up

1. Introduction

Over 12,400 children and adolescents younger than 20 years of age are diagnosed with cancer in the United States every year [1]. Survival for many pediatric cancers has improved significantly in the past three decades with improvement in therapies. The surveillance, epidemiology, and end results data estimate that the overall five-year survival rate among children for all cancer sites combined improved from 58% for patients diagnosed in 1975–1977 to 80% for those diagnosed in 1996–2003 [1].

There were an estimated 388,501 survivors of childhood cancer in the United States as of January 1, 2011, of whom 83.5% are ≥5 years after diagnosis [2]. Frequently, long-term survivors of childhood cancer report late cancer-related effects that diminish quality of life and persisting after cancer treatment may result in premature onset of common diseases associated with aging such as obesity, diabetes mellitus, cardiovascular disease, hypertension, and second cancers [3–5].

Risk-based health care that involves a personalized plan for surveillance, screening, and prevention is recommended to reduce cancer-related morbidity in childhood cancer survivors. However, there are few consensus recommendations and very few specialized centers providing this care. Moreover, to implement this model, the survivor and healthcare provider must have accurate information about cancer diagnosis, treatment modalities, and potential cancer-related health risks to guide screening and risk-reducing interventions. Childhood Cancer Survivor Study (CCSS) data show that approximately half of the approximately 14,000 responding long-term survivors of childhood cancer had not been seen by a physician during the previous 2 years for evaluation of cancer-related problems. A recent survey of Pediatric Oncology Group and Children's Cancer Group member sites reported that 44% of the sites have a mechanism for following adult survivors, but only 15% of the programs have a formal database for these patients [6].

In this chapter, we describe the common late effects based on therapy received for cancer and provide the current evidence regarding guidelines available for long-term follow-up of pediatric cancer survivors. We also address the lacunas in patient and physician education and current evidence regarding interventions to address this to improve the quality of life for pediatric cancer survivors.

2. Late effects of cancer therapy

Late effects are those toxicities related to therapy for cancer that are absent or subclinical at the end of therapy but manifest later. Compensatory mechanisms that initially maintain the function of injured organs may fail with growth, development, and aging. We discuss below the common late effects of cancer chemotherapy in children. **Table 1** summarizes the most common late effects in survivors of childhood cancer. **Tables 2** and **3** summarize some of the common late effects and screening methodology used to monitor and manage them.

2.1. Mortality

Type and intensity of therapy as well as the patient's age at therapy determine not only the overall survival but also the frequency of late effects of cancer therapy [7]. Some studies have shown excessive mortality rates in five-year survivors of childhood cancer [8–12]. The Childhood Cancer Survivor Study (CCSS), a retrospective cohort study initiated in 1994, was

http://dx.doi.org/10.5772/67366

Adverse event category
Alopecia
Ear, nose, and throat
Fatigue
Pain
Pulmonary
Tissue hypoplasia
Urology
Miscellaneous
Ophthalmology
Gastroenterology
Cardiovascular
Angina pectoris/Myocardial infarction
Cardiomyopathy
Nephrologic
Hypertension
Tubular dysfunction
Orthopedic
Amputation/Prothesis/Rotationplasty
Scoliosis/Low back pain
Psychosocial/Cognitive problems
Cognitive problems
Emotional problems
Fertility
Oligospermia/Azoospermia
Metabolic
Obesity
Second tumors
Malignant
Endocrine
Growth hormone deficiency
Thyroid disorders
Panhypopituitarism
Neurologic
Seizures
Motor dysfunction/Hemiparesis
Sensory loss

Table 1. Common adverse events in a cohort of childhood cancer survivors.

Organ	Therapy	Screening test
Musculoskeletal	Radiotherapy(RT)	Physical exam scoliosis exam (annually if growing), X-ray pm
Breast	Mediastinal RT	Breast exam. mammography beginning age 25–30
CNS	Cranial RT	Neurocognitive testing (baseline, q 3-5 yrs pm). MRI (baseline)
Neuroendocrine	Hypothala/mic-pituitary RT	Growm curve q yr. bone age (age 9)
		GH stimulation test
		TSH, Free T4.T3 (baseline q 3-5 yr pm)
		LH FSH. test/est. prolactin (baseline, pm)
		8 am cortisol (baseline, pm)
Cardiac	Anthracyclines mediastinal T-spine RT	ECHO'EKG (baseline for all; q 3-5 yr after anthracycline) Holter q 5 yrs pm (high-dose anthracycline) Stress test/ dobutamine stress echo pm (after RT)
Pulmonary	RT	PFT baseline, q 3-5 yrs pm
	Bleomycin, CCNU/BCNU	
Ovary	Alkylating agents	Menstrual 'Hx annually
	RT	LH FSH estradiol baseline (age>12) and pm
Testes	Alkylating agents	LH FSH. testos baseline (age >12) and pm
	RT	Spermatoanalysis pm
Renal	Cisplatin (carboplatin),	Creatinine, Mg, q 1-2 yrs
	Ifosfamide,	Ceatinine clearance baseline and q 3-5 yrs pm
	RT	Urinalysis (RT. ifosfamide)
		Ifosfamide: serum phosphate. urine glucose, protein
Bladder	Cyclophosphamide,	Urinalysis annually for heme
	Ifosfamide. RT	
Thyroid	RT to neck, mediastinum	TSH, FreeT4,T3q yr X 10
		Scans (U/S) pm
Liner	6-MP,MTX,Act-d, RT	Liver function tests every 1–3 years
GI	Intestinal RT	Stool guiac q yr, colonoscopy (ACS)

Table 2. Example of screening methodology for late effects specific to treatment received.

designed to study late effects among long-term survivors of childhood cancer. It showed a 10.8-fold excess in overall mortality. Risk of death was significantly higher in females, those with an initial diagnosis of leukemia or brain tumor and those diagnosed with cancer before they turned 5 years old. Sixty percent of deaths were from recurrence of the original cancer that was the leading cause of death. Statistically significant excess mortality rates were seen due to various causes shown in **Table 4**. Treatment-related associations were reported for cancer mortality (radiation, epipodophyllotoxins, alkylating agents), cardiac mortality (chest irradiation), and other deaths (radiation, anthracyclines). No excess mortality was seen for external causes [13].

http://dx.doi.org/10.5772/67366

Chemotherapy		
If patient received:		
Actinomycin or antimetabolite	ALT	Periodically
	Bone densitometry	Optional
Aminogtycoside, high dose	Audiology	Optional
Anthracycline	Echocardiogram	Every 3 years
(≥300 mg/m², or anthracycline administered prior to age 1 year	EKG	Optional
or ≥200 mg/m² with radiation involving the chest)		
BCNU, CCNIl, bleoraycin	CXR	Baseline
	Pulmonary function tests	Baseline and as needed
Cisplatin	BUN, creatinine, magnesium	Annually
	Audiology	Optional
Corticosteroids	Bone deisitometry	Optional
Cyclophosphamide	FSH, LH, estradiol	Optional
	Semen analysis	Optional
	Urinalysis	Annually
	Urine cytology	Optional
Cyclosporine	Bone densitometry	Optional
Etoposide	CBC with platelets and differential	Annually
Nitrogen mustard, procarbazine	CBC with platelets and differential	Annually
	FSH, LH, estradiol	Optional
	Testosterone	Optional
	Semen analysis	Optional
Vinciistine	ALT	Periodically
Radiation therapy		
If patient received;		
Cranial or craniospinal radiation	Cataract screening	Periodically
	Audiology	Optional
	Dental screening	Annually
	TSH, Free T_4	Annually
	Lipid profile	Annually
	Bone densitometry	Optional
Mande radiation	TSH	Annually
	Lipid profile	Annually

	Mammogram (females)	Start 8 years after radiation, then annually
	Plain radiographs of irradiated site	Optional
Abdominal radiation	Hernoccult screening	Annually
	Urinalysis	Annually
Pehic radiation	FSH.LH	Optional
	Semen analysis	Optional
High-dose radiation of the Hunk or extremities	Plain radiographs of the irradiated sites	Optional
Surgery		
If patient received:		
Nephrectomy	BUN, creatinine, urinalysis	Annually
Splenectomy	Verify immunizations	Annually
	Antibiotic prophvlaxis	Optional

Table 3. Organ-specific late effects of cancer therapy and screening methodology.

-Recurrence
-Treatment-related consequences
Subsequent neoplasm
Lip, oral cavity, pharynx, lung
Digestive organs and peritoneum
Bone and articular cartilage
Connective and other soft tissue
Melanoma and other skin
Breast
Genitourinary organs
Brain and other parts of nervous system
Lymphatic and hematopoietic
Other subsequent cancer
Cardiac
Ischemic heart disease
Cardiomyopathy
Congestive heart failure
Other cardiac
Pulmonary

Pulmonary fibrosis
Other pulmonary
Other sequelae
Infectious disease
Other sequelae
-Nontreatment-related causes of death
External causes
Motor vehicle accident
Other accident
Suicide
Homicide
Medical conditions
Human immunodeficiency virus
Pneumonia
Other bacterial/viral infection
Heart disease
Cerebrovascular disease
Other medical condition

Table 4. Specific causes of mortality in Childhood Cancer Survivor Study cohort.

2.2. Growth and development

The effects on growth and development are dependent on dose and the developmental process of the organ in question. Therapy for the treatment of malignancy may interfere with development in terms of physical growth, neurocognitive growth, musculoskeletal growth (hypoplasia), and, ultimately, pubertal development.

2.3. Physical growth

Growth is often impaired in children with active cancer and those undergoing intense therapies due to hypermetabolic states, the effects of chronic disease, and poor nutrition. After the completion of therapy, many children experience a growth spurt and normalization of growth but specific therapies may interfere with this [14].

2.3.1. Hypoplasia

Localized radiotherapy affects skin and musculoskeletal growth causing cosmetic concern in radiation-treated survivors. Asymmetric radiation fields result in differential growth of the radiated versus nonirradiated tissue. Functional effects, such as muscle or back pain due to radiation-induced scoliosis, can occur. Hypoplasia is not apparent at the end of therapy but becomes manifest with growth, particularly during the pubertal spurt. Particular sensitivity of adipose tissue to radiation may lead to asymmetric fat distribution with weight gain any time in life. Breast asymmetry occurs after unilateral chest radiotherapy prior to maturity. Doses of 20 Gy may stop breast development completely, whereas 10 Gy to the breast bud may cause hypoplasia [15, 16]. Lactation may not be possible for women [17].

2.3.2. *Linear growth effects*

Cranial irradiation affects linear growth by its effect on the hypothalamic-pituitary axis. The effect is dependent on dose and age. Patients treated with large doses of whole brain radiotherapy are likely to have growth hormone deficiency requiring hormone replacement. Growth velocity after lower doses of radiotherapy may proceed normally until puberty, at which time the classic "growth spurt" may be impaired [18]. Early onset of puberty is common after cranial radiation, reducing final height [18] and this effect is more pronounced if the child is younger at the time of radiation [19]. Childhood cancer survivors treated with cranial radiation may have a higher body mass index [20], which is inversely related to the age of puberty [21, 22]. After spinal radiotherapy, the effect of aberrant growth hormone release and early puberty may be worsened by vertebral stature loss after spinal irradiation [23]. These effects can be mitigated prior to closure of the epiphyses. Close monitoring of growth is needed but may not be sufficient. The role of growth hormone stimulation beginning shortly after completion of therapy and inhibition of the pubertal spurt to prolong the potential growth phase is being assessed [19].

2.3.3. *Intellectual development*

Intellectual outcome after the completion of therapy is important for integration successfully into society after completion of therapy. Central nervous system (CNS) radiotherapy or high-dose chemotherapy that achieves sufficient CNS levels for the prevention of meningeal leukemia may result in cognitive deficits [24]. Impairment of memory, attention, and visual perceptual motor skills result in problems with language, reading, and arithmetic and poor academic achievement [24, 25]. Brain injury may become more apparent years after the completion of therapy and intellectual growth suffers over time [26]. The severity of the effect is determined by both dose of therapy and the time at which it was given. Higher doses [>36 Gy] have significant deficits that virtually always require special educational efforts [27]. Cognitive effects of radiation on infant development are profound and hence high doses may be deferred until after age two [27]. Preschool children receiving doses in the range of 18–24 Gy of cranial radiotherapy often require special educational resources, and older children may have difficulties with complex systems such as a new language or high-level mathematics [27]. At lower doses of radiation, children are likely to remain within the mainstream education efforts but may need help to achieve maximal success. Significant doses of intrathecal chemotherapy may have similar effects [27]. Most survivors enter college at the same rates as siblings, except for those receiving 24 Gy or treated as preschoolers; however, an overall need for special education exists and occupational success may not be equal to that of siblings [28].

http://dx.doi.org/10.5772/67366

2.4. Organ specific effects

2.4.1. Gonadal toxicity and pubertal development

It is tough to clinically assess the extent of treatment-induced gonadal damage suffered during childhood. Anticipatory guidance can be given based upon reported experience. Close monitoring throughout puberty is vital as initial pubertal development may proceed even with severe gonadal injury as a result of adrenal corticoid hormones. Long delays in assessment may have severe social consequences.

Alkylating agents are known for inducing infertility; little gonadal toxicity is noted after the antimetabolites, vinca alkaloids, anthracyclines, bleomycin, or platinum derivatives. Sertoli cells are more sensitive than Leydig cells to radiation and alkylating agents [29, 30]. Young boys may proceed with normal masculinization, potency, and libido even with azoospermia due to preservation of Leydig cells. Testosterone levels as well as pubertal development should be assessed for recipients of high-dose chemotherapy. By late puberty, testosterone deficiency should be treated to normalize masculinization. Even though ovaries are less sensitive than testes to gonadotoxic agents [30, 31], an affected female child may experience pubertal delay and amenorrhea. Hormone replacement to preserve feminization and periods may be needed. Another reason for treating estradiol deficiency is the prevention of osteoporosis and early coronary artery disease. Cranial radiation at higher doses can also result in secondary gonadal insufficiency by impairment in LH/FSH production and secretion. In those brain tumor patients receiving hypothalamic-pituitary axis radiation as well as alkylating agents (e.g., BCNU, CCNU), direct gonadal effects as well as secondary gonadal insufficiency are seen [31].

Reversibility is dependent on dose of gonadal radiation or alkylating agents. Ovarian function is unlikely to recover long after the immediate therapy due to loss of ova. The testis is more sensitive to cytotoxic therapies than the ovary, but late recovery (2–12 years after radiotherapy) has been reported [32]. Prediction of fertility in an adult woman may be indicated by evaluation of her menstrual cycle. The same dose of drug is more likely to affect an older woman than a younger one [33]. Although young women may not become amenorrheic after cytotoxic therapy, the risk of early menopause exists. Direct radiotherapy to the ovaries also causes infertility. Oophoropexy is commonly offered to prevent infertility in women whose ovaries would otherwise remain in the radiation field. Lower doses or even scatter of radiation within the small body of an infant or toddler may have profound effects. Oophoropexy is not an option in this population since the small torso does not offer a sanctuary for the ovaries. Flank radiotherapy such as for Wilms' tumor does not affect the ovaries but may result in reduced fetal size by effects on the uterine muscle and vasculature [34, 35].

Male sterility is usual after approximately 10 g/m^2 of cyclophosphamide. The prepubertal state offers, at best, only limited protection to testes treated with cyclophosphamide [36]. Ten percent of men will become sterile after one to two cycles of MOPP chemotherapy commonly used in Hodgkin's disease in the past, while 80–100% are sterile after six courses [36]. Low doses (2–3 Gy) of radiotherapy result in azoospermia in all males, with late recovery noted occasionally after a period of years.

New reproductive technologies have improved outcomes for infertile cancer survivors. Sperm banking, the ability to inseminate ova with only small numbers of spermatozoa, and artificial insemination are the most frequently used approaches for sterile male survivors. Female survivors have more limited options. Storage of ova is being researched actively [37].

Hyperprolactinemia is another easily treatable and fairly common but often missed effect of hypothalamic-pituitary irradiation that may impair fertility as well as growth and libido [38]. Appropriate endocrinologic interventions with dopamine agonists can be helpful.

2.4.2. Cardiac

Anthracyclines are important in the treatment of most childhood cancers. Unfortunately, cardiac damage is most pronounced after treatment with anthracyclines, with additive effects of cyclophosphamide and radiation therapy. Anthracyclines cause decrease in myocyte number by causing myocardial cell death. Residual myocytes hypertrophy in a compensatory manner [39]. Cardiac injury during or shortly after the completion of chemotherapy may progress, stabilize, or improve after the first year [40]. Patients with reduced cardiac function within 6 months of completing chemotherapy are at increased risk for the development of late cardiac failure [41].

Myocardial injury can be detected with sensitive screening tests, even after a cumulative dose of 45 mg/m^2 [42, 43]. Unfortunately, these tests are not routinely available. Initial improvement in cardiac function from compensatory changes may diminish with later stressors in life. For example, myocardial depressants such as alcohol or increased afterload brought on by exercise, growth spurts, or pregnancy may induce late cardiac failure. Isometric exercise may increase the risk for late cardiac failure, particularly in after neck or mantle radiotherapy [44]. There is evidence to suggest that there is a continuum of injury that will manifest itself throughout the lives of these patients [45]. Many pediatric cardiologists may advise patients to avoid excessive alcohol intake and isometric exercises such as weight-lifting. Those who have received the higher doses of anthracyclines need the closest monitoring and counseling.

Pregnancy, a time of increased cardiac demand, is a dangerous period for anthracycline-treated women. These women need to be evaluated by a cardiologist. Obstetricians should be made aware that these women may have limited ability to compensate for the increased cardiac output of pregnancy. Careful monitoring during pregnancy and the postpartum period is essential. Women with significantly limited cardiac reserve may be advised that pregnancy may carry unacceptable risk [44].

Severe cardiac effects of radiation may be noted including valvular damage, pericardial thickening, and ischemic heart disease [46]. Patients have an increased risk of both angina and myocardial infarction years after radiotherapy for Hodgkin's disease [47], with a relative risk of 3.1 for cardiac death with Hodgkin's disease [48]. This risk was noted in those receiving >30 Gy of mantle irradiation and was greatest for those treated before 20 years of age [49]. The use of anteriorly weighted ports, reduction in total tumor and daily fraction dose, and cardiac shielding are some of the techniques being used to reduce the effects of radiation [49].

2.4.3. Pulmonary

The effects of chemotherapy on the lungs may be lethal or may improve gradually. However, pulmonary function tests may not return to normal, and there may be slow clinical decline. Long-term outcome depends on severity of the acute injury, the extent of compensation, and the likelihood of decompensation. It is reported that 35% of children treated for brain tumors with nitrosourea and radiotherapy died of pulmonary fibrosis, 12% within 3 years and 24% after a symptom-free period of 7–12 years [50]. Therefore, the recommended dose limit of nitrosourea's in children has been lowered from 1500 to 750 mg/m^2 but the late effects of this lower dose need to be assessed [50]. Some chemotherapy drugs like cyclophosphamide when used orally may cause restrictive lung disease by inhibition of chest wall growth. This effect may become apparent as late as 7 years after the completion of therapy [51]. It has not been reported after modern intravenous cyclophosphamide regimens. Patients treated with bleomycin may experience pulmonary insufficiency from interstitial pneumonitis characterized by a reticulo-nodular pattern [52, 53]. Even after the completion of therapy, the risk for overt decompensation remains for at least 1 year. A recent study by Kung et al. has noted that 22% of Hodgkin's disease patients with normal pulmonary function tests at the end of therapy developed abnormalities with follow-up of 1–7 years [54, 55]. In long-term follow-up, pulmonary dysfunction is usually subclinical. Subconscious avoidance of exercise is rarely attributed to therapy or recognized by the patient himself. Patients who have been treated with pulmonary radiation and cytotoxic agents such as BCNU, CCNU, and bleomycin should undergo pulmonary function testing every 5–8 years [56]. Such patients should avoid exposure to pulmonary toxins, most notably cigarettes. Radiation itself (>9 Gy) raised the risk of lung cancer after Hodgkin's disease.

2.4.4. Genitourinary tract

The most commonly noted renal problems after radiation therapy, especially with doses greater than 20 Gy are tubular damage and hypertension associated with renal artery stenosis [57, 58]. Children may be susceptible to these complications at lower doses. In addition, chemotherapy may exacerbate these effects [59]. Chemotherapy alone, particularly platinum compounds are notorious for glomerular and tubular injury [60, 61]. Glomerular injury may recover over time, while tubular injury persists. The nitrosourea may affect glomerular function. Ifosfamide results in renal Fanconi's syndrome with glycosuria, phosphaturia, and aminoaciduria [62]. Hypophosphatemia may result in slow growth and bone disease. Glomerular filtration may also be affected by ifosfamide. In children, there is a risk of renal decompensation with growth with any of these injuries. The bladder is susceptible to cytotoxic agents such as cyclophosphamide and ifosfamide that have acrolein as a by-product. Acrolein may result hemorrhage cystitis, fibrosis, diminished bladder volume, and rarely bladder cancer [63–65]. Patients who have received one of these agents should have an annual urinalysis, with further evaluation if hematuria is noted. Radiation may induce bladder fibrosis, decreasing contractibility and decreased volume depending on dose and area exposed [66]. Scarring may also diminish function of the urethra and ureter.

2.4.5. *Thyroid gland*

Damage to thyroid is common after radiotherapy to the neck and chest. Patients treated for Hodgkin's disease in whom the thyroid was irradiated had a 47% risk of overt or compensated hypothyroidism at 26 years [67]. Although compensatory increase in thyroid-stimulating hormone (TSH) initially maintains the euthyroid clinical state, further deterioration of thyroid function often results in clinical symptomatology. Treatment with thyroid hormone is recommended with persistent evidence of compensated hypothyroidism. Chronically elevated TSH levels in the presence of irradiated thyroid tissue can enhance tumor development [68, 69]. Benign nodules, Graves' disease, thyroid cancer, and Hashimoto's thyroiditis are some of the other disorders seen after radiation to the gland [67].

2.4.6. *Gastrointestinal/hepatic*

There is not much literature describing long-term effects to this system. This may be due to long latency of the late effects or under detection. Many chemotherapeutic agents as well as radiotherapy may be damaging to the liver; therefore, it may be difficult to attribute the harm to specific therapy. Transfusions increase the risk of viral hepatitis. Hepatitis C has been identified in increasing numbers of survivors [70]. Fibrosis and adhesions of bowel are known to occur after radiotherapy.

2.4.7. *Second malignancies*

About 4% of survivors develop a secondary malignancy within 25 years of diagnosis of the primary cancer [71]. This is an excess risk of six times among survivors compared to healthy individuals and is contributed to by the carcinogenic effects of treatments for the original childhood cancer as well as to genetic predisposition [71]. Bone cancers, mostly osteosarcomas, are the most common solid second cancers observed after all types of childhood cancer other than retinoblastoma [72, 73]. There is probably some element of genetic predisposition, which would include, for example, constitutional mutations of the p53 gene that contributes to secondary cancers after childhood cancers [74, 75]. Second primary leukemia is diagnosed in about 0.2% of survivors of childhood cancer within 6 years of diagnosis of the original cancer—about eight times the expected number of leukemia [76].

2.4.8. *Education, psychosocial, and quality of life issues*

Evidence suggests that survivors of childhood cancer experienced a range of educational, behavioral, and social problems. The extent of problems experienced varies by the disease and its treatment, as well as by demographic and family variables [77, 78]. Children miss substantial amounts of schooling during treatment, and this affects both academic achievement and social relationships. Fairly consistent evidence shows that intrathecal chemotherapy and radiotherapy to the CNS impacts academic achievement and learning. Children under 5 years at diagnosis are particularly vulnerable. A general decline in intellectual function or deficits in specific skills, including attention, concentration, and mathematical reasoning may be seen [79, 80]. Measurement of social function is more complex than measurement of academic function, and perhaps for this reason there is limited literature describing social functioning among survivors. Among children of school age, there is some evidence that survivors of a central nervous system tumor are less popular with other children [81]. Many survivors need appropriate and sensitive counseling to enable them to choose and succeed in appropriate employment [82]. There is a considerable variation in quality of life among survivors [82]. Several studies report compromises in mental health among survivors [82].

3. Prevention of late effects

Several agents designed to protect normal tissues from the toxic effects of specific therapeutic agents are being evaluated. Examples of these agents include amifostine (cisplatinum-induced ototoxicity) [83] and dexrazoxane (anthracycline-induced cardiomyopathy) [84]. Long-term follow-up will be required to assess the efficacy of all these strategies. Research related to determination of whether agents used to protect normal tissues will or slow down the progression of an adverse late effect, is less well developed. Specific research initiatives include the use of afterload reducing agents for prevention of further progression of myocardial dysfunction [85], use of chemoprevention for prevention of secondary malignancies, lifestyle and behavior modification, and education to increase awareness of the need for screening for early detection.

3.1. Guidelines for follow-up of pediatric cancer survivors

Awareness of the potential health problems as a result of treatment for cancer in childhood is less than optimal among practitioners and survivors themselves. In contrast to the multitude of publications describing treatment-related sequelae in childhood cancer survivors, relatively few provide specific recommendations for health screening and risk-reduction counseling to guide healthcare providers in monitoring this vulnerable population [5, 86–90]. To reach this goal, several barriers need to be surpassed, notably education of survivors and healthcare providers regarding the late effects of cancer treatment; availability of standardized guidelines for follow-up of the survivors in a feasible and practical setting and ongoing communication between the cancer center that provided acute care for the patient and the facility providing follow-up care. Among the hurdles to guideline development are ongoing changes in pediatric cancer therapy, long latency periods required to evaluate many late effects, the unknown effects of aging, and the multiple factors known to influence cancer-related health risks in patients who received cancer therapy during childhood [86, 91]. Despite these challenges, two sets of clinical follow-up guidelines designed to guide care for pediatric cancer survivors have recently been published and are described below.

3.1.1. Children's Oncology Group (COG) Long-Term Follow-up (LTFU) Guidelines

The COG is a 242-member National Cancer Institute-supported cooperative clinical trials group whose goals include minimizing the risk of long-term effects that may impact duration and/or quality of life in pediatric cancer survivors. COG recently developed risk-based, exposure-related guidelines (Long-Term Follow-up Guidelines for Survivors of Childhood,

Adolescent, and Young Adult Cancers] for use in directing follow-up care for survivors of pediatric malignancies [86].

The COG-LTFU Guidelines are risk-based, exposure-related clinical practice guidelines for screening and management of late effects resulting from therapeutic exposures used during the treatment of pediatric malignancies. The guidelines are both evidence-based and based on the collective clinical experience of experts (matching the magnitude of the risk with the intensity of the screening recommendations). The screening recommendations are provided in these guidelines area consensus statement from a panel of experts in the late effects of pediatric cancer treatment. A therapy-based design was chosen to permit formatting of the guidelines by therapeutic exposure since the therapeutic interventions for a specific pediatric malignancy may differ considerably based on the patient's age, presenting features, and treatment era [86]. The guidelines are therefore organized according to therapeutic agent, and cross-referenced to other topics with related toxicities. The guidelines are designed to standardize and direct follow-up care that facilitates early identification of and intervention for treatment-related complications. Limitations include the potential for false-positive screening evaluations and increased patient anxiety related to an increased awareness of possible complications. Costs of long-term follow-up care may also be prohibitive for some patients.

Goal of implementation of these guidelines is to increase quality of life and decrease complication-related healthcare costs for pediatric cancer survivors by providing standardized and enhanced follow-up care throughout the life span. The guidelines are intended for use beginning 2 or more years following the completion of cancer therapy to [1] promote healthy lifestyles [2], provide ongoing monitoring of health status [3], facilitate early identification of late effects, and [4] provide timely intervention for late effects. The information within these guidelines is important for clinicians (e.g., physicians, nurse practitioners, physician assistants, nurses) in the fields of pediatrics, oncology, internal medicine, family practice, and gynecology, as well as subspecialists in many fields (e.g., endocrinology, cardiology, pulmonology) [86]. **Figure 1** presents an example model of how these guidelines were developed.

3.1.2. SIGN guidelines

The goal of Scottish Intercollegiate Guidelines Network (SIGN) is to develop evidence-based clinical guidelines aimed at reducing variations in clinical practice and outcomes for patients [91]. SIGN is composed of members from all medical specialties, nursing, pharmacy, dentistry, allied health professionals, patients, health service managers, social services, and researchers [91]. SIGN recently developed national guidelines for pediatric cancer survivors (SIGN guidelines) [91].The SIGN guideline provides a detailed review of the following topics with evidence for each and grading for each recommendation and its rationale: (1) assessment and achievement of normal growth; (2) achievement of normal progression through puberty and factors affecting fertility; (3) early identification, assessment and treatment of cardiac abnormalities; (4) assessment of thyroid function; and 5] assessment and achievement of optimum neurodevelopment and psychological

http://dx.doi.org/10.5772/67366

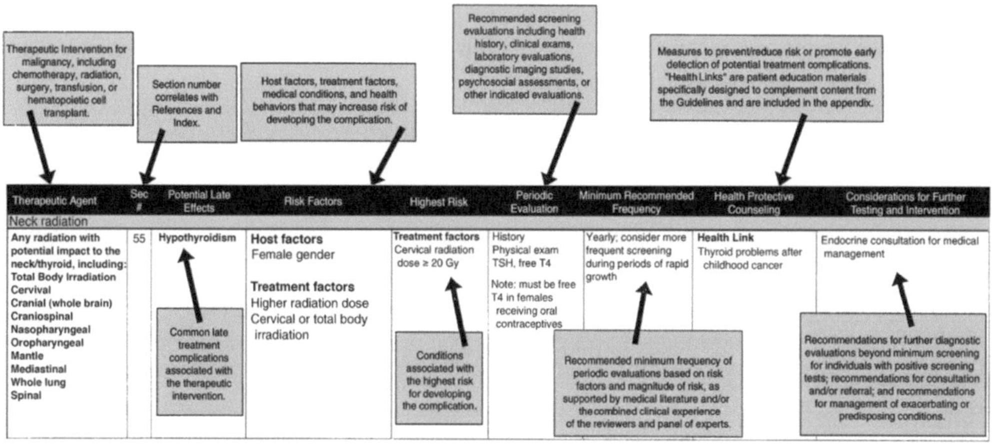

Figure 1. Sample excerpt from the Children's Oncology Group Long-Term Follow-Up Guidelines for survivors of childhood, adolescent, and young adult cancers. TSH, thyroid-stimulating hormone.

health [92, 93]. Limitations of the SIGN guideline include lack of specific follow-up recommendations for areas such as renal, pulmonary, gastrointestinal, ocular, auditory, and musculoskeletal systems as well as second malignancies. In addition to clinical recommendations, the SIGN guideline contains recommendations for the delivery of follow-up care for pediatric cancer survivors, based on the intensity of treatment received. The degree of long-term risk is determined by site of the underlying malignancy, type and intensity of treatment, and age of patient at treatment. Three levels of follow-up are described: "Level 1" follow-up is suggested for those survivors for whom the benefit of clinical follow-up is not clearly established. Annual or even every two-year postal or telephone contact is recommended. "Level 2" follow-up is suggested for the majority of patients on current protocols. Nurse or primary care follow-up on an annual basis may suffice. "Level 3" follow-up is for patients who have received radiotherapy, bone marrow transplantation, or megatherapy, and who have a significant risk of long-term morbidity [92, 93]. Recommendations for these patients include follow-up in a medically supervised long-term follow-up clinic three to four times per year [92, 93].

3.1.3. *Application of guidelines to clinical practice*

The main challenge of providing quality care to a pediatric cancer survivor is combining routine age-appropriate health maintenance with exposure-related screening for potential late-onset complications related to pediatric cancer therapy. Ideally, evaluations should be individualized based on the survivor's treatment history. A balance between over-screening, which might induce anxiety related to unlikely complications, and under-screening for potentially life-threatening complications that if missed at an early phase may require more aggressive intervention later needs to be achieved. Screening guidelines that can be individualized based on the patient's risk for developing a particular complication are therefore ideal. As the COG and SIGN guidelines become more widely implemented over time, refinements will undoubtedly be made that will make them even more clinically relevant and practical for survivors who are followed in future years.

The importance of educating both survivor and healthcare professionals about potential late effects cannot be over-emphasized since a wide range of providers are involved in the follow-up of these patients including nurses, psychologists, social workers, adult and pediatric primary care providers, and specialists in many fields. Ultimately, as with all clinical practice guidelines, decisions regarding implementation of specific screening modalities and ongoing clinical management should be tailored to individual patients, taking into consideration all relevant factors, including medical and psychosocial history, therapeutic exposures, risk factors, and co-morbidities [93].

3.1.4. Limitations in providing long-term follow-up care

3.1.4.1. Patient factors

Misperceptions about their cancer diagnosis, treatment, and cancer-related health risks exist among cancer survivors [94–96]. Byrne et al. [90] surveyed 1928 adult survivors of childhood cancer diagnosed between 1945 and 1974 to assess knowledge of their cancer diagnosis. Overall, 14% of survivors were not aware that they had cancer. Lesser knowledge of their diagnosis was associated with younger age at treatment, nonwhite race, less intensive treatment, and lower parental education status. It is possible that racial, socioeconomic, and cultural factors that were prevalent during the period when the patient was diagnosed may influence the interaction amongst the oncologist and patient [90]. Historically, some healthcare professionals and families prefer giving limited information about cancer-related health risk to survivors due to concerns about inducing anxiety. In a similar study from 1970 to 1986, Childhood Cancer Survivor Study (CCSS) investigators evaluated the accuracy of self-reported information acquired from a cross-sectional survey of 635 adult survivors of childhood cancer. Knowledge about cancer history and its associated health risks is improved in more recently treated survivors compared to the Byrne study [94]. More than 90% of participants were aware of their cancer diagnosis but not all elements of their history in a recent study. The knowledge deficits about cancer-related health risks in older survivors may limit their participation in screening and risk-reducing programs [97].

3.1.4.2. Provider factors

Healthcare providers encountering childhood cancer survivors must be knowledgeable about potential cancer-related adverse effects in order to prescribe appropriate monitoring and interventions should health problems arise. Because of the rarity and complexity of numerous histologic subtypes with unique epidemiology, biology, and treatment regimens managing long-term childhood cancer survivors is an intimidating task for primary care physicians. Healthcare providers are unlikely to care for more than a handful of survivors, usually each with different cancers, treatment exposures, and health risks making it difficult to attain proficiency. Consequently, primary healthcare providers in the community are often uncomfortable with supervising the care of childhood cancer survivors.

The knowledge, attitudes, and beliefs of physicians providing care for survivors of childhood cancer have not been well studied. Several investigators coordinating late effects surveyed a convenience sample of 236 physicians from around the United States, in private or academic practices using a 36-item questionnaire that asked about knowledge, attitudes, and beliefs in providing health care for adult survivors of childhood cancer [98]. In comparison with pediatric oncologists, primary care physicians (general internists and family physicians) reported a lower level of knowledge regarding both common childhood cancers and the late effects with treatment exposures. A recent study in the UK reported a cross-sectional postal survey as well as a cross-sectional postal survey of general practitioners of 10,979 adult survivors of childhood cancer in Britain. This study has shown that there are wide variations in the extent to which survivors of childhood cancer are discharged from hospital follow-up [99]. Adult oncologists generally reported a higher level of knowledge of these factors than primary care physicians, but considerably less than pediatric oncologists. Notably, primary care physicians expressed a lower level of comfort in managing survivors. These data point to a need for resources and interventions that specifically address the unique needs and medical management of childhood cancer survivors that primary care providers might benefit from.

3.1.5. Solutions for coordinated care for childhood cancer survivors

3.1.5.1. Specialized long-term follow-up clinics

Multidisciplinary long-term follow-up teams at some pediatric oncology treatment centers have established long-term follow-up clinics. Follow-up in this model is limited to an annual comprehensive multidisciplinary health evaluation, and survivors are encouraged to establish an ongoing relationship with a primary healthcare provider in the community for routine health maintenance. Benefits of this approach are that the patient remains in contact with a team that is knowledgeable and has a standardized program of long-term follow-up care, contact with the original treatment center is maintained, and multidisciplinary referrals available within the healthcare system. Disadvantages include the lack of familiarity of the pediatric treatment team with age related health-care issues that might arise, reluctance of the older patient to return to a pediatric facility, reimbursement for specialized services not covered by insurance companies, and problems of access due to long distances between the medical center and the survivor's residence [100].

3.1.5.2. Transition models

In some instances, institutions have established formalized transition programs with specialized long-term follow-up programs for adult survivors of childhood cancer because of reluctance of pediatric oncology centers to take care of adult cancer survivors. Transition programs may utilize both oncology and primary care providers in a collaborative framework, and maintain many of the benefits of the specialized long-term follow-up clinics, with the benefit of care providers with expertise in adult medicine. One limitation is that since the focus is on survivorship care, and ongoing primary care is often not accessible through these specialized programs, and distance to the center may remain a barrier [100].

3.1.5.3. Transition to adult oncology

In this model, when the survivor reaches adulthood, the pediatric provider makes a referral to an adult oncologist for ongoing follow-up. Advantages of this system include ongoing monitoring for disease recurrence in an adult medical care system, and accessibility to care in the local community. Disadvantages include the limited familiarity of most adult oncologists with the potential late complications of chemotherapy and radiotherapy in children and the appropriate follow-up evaluations indicated for childhood cancer survivors [100].

3.1.5.4. Community-based care

Follow-up care may be provided by an adult primary care provider (e.g., internist, family practitioner), who maintains communication with the original pediatric oncology treatment team. Advantages of this model include ability to maintain a relationship with a provider in the community who is familiar with their specialized healthcare needs and disadvantages include the primary care provider's lack of familiarity with potential late effects. There may also be limited access to multidisciplinary specialty care providers that many survivors require [100].

4. Conclusions

As pediatric oncologists, our work is not done when the cancer is cured. We must try to recognize, monitor and decrease the late effects of cancer therapy when possible and, if not possible, to understand the effects so that future treatment regimens can be designed with less risks of late effects. Remarkable improvement in cure rates has been achieved by persistent stress on designing effective therapy. Only by continued, systematic follow-up of large cohorts of survivors will we know the full spectrum of damage caused by cytotoxic therapy and possible interventions that may mitigate the effects. Ongoing methods for educating both the patient and the primary caretakers must be devised. We must set up programs to evaluate the survivors to assess and care for chronic organ damage, providing the necessary support for the primary physician. As part of a collaborative effort, the primary care provider and the specialist must work toward the goal of best possible quality of life for the pediatric cancer survivor.

Author details

Nupur Mittal[1]* and Paul Kent[2]

*Address all correspondence to: nupur_mittal@rush.edu

1 Department of Pediatrics, Rush Medical College, Chicago, IL, United States

2 Division of Pediatric Hematology/Oncology, Department of Pediatrics, Rush University Medical Center, Chicago, IL, United States

References

[1] Ries LAG, Smith MA, Gurney JG, et al., eds. Cancer incidence and survival among children and adolescents: United States SEER Program 1975–1995. National Cancer Institute, SEER Program. Bethesda, MD, NIH Publication No. 99–4649, 1999.

[2] Phillips SM, Padgett LS, Leisenring WM et al. Survivors of childhood cancer in the United States: Prevalence and burden of morbidity. Cancer Epidemiol Biomarkers Prev 2015 Apr;24[4]:653–663. doi: 10.1158/1055-9965.EPI-14-1418.

[3] Neglia JP, Friedman DL, Yasui Y, et al. Second malignant neoplasms in five-year survivors of childhood cancer: Childhood cancer survivor study. J Natl Cancer Inst 2001;93:618–629.

[4] Hudson MM, Poquette CA, Lee J, et al. Increased mortality after successful treatment for Hodgkin's disease. J Clin Oncol 1998;16:3592–3600.

[5] Green DM, Hyland A, Chung CS, et al. Cancer and cardiac mortality among 15-year survivors of cancer diagnosed during childhood or adolescence. J Clin Oncol 1999;17: 3207–3215.

[6] Oeffinger KC, Eshelman DA, Tomlinson GE, Buchanan GR. Programs for adult survivors of childhood cancer. J ClinOncol 1998;16:2864–2867.

[7] Oeffinger KC[1], Eshelman DA, Tomlinson GE. Grading of late effects in young adult survivors of childhood cancer followed in an ambulatory adult setting. Cancer. 2000 Apr 1;88[7]:1687–1695.

[8] Hudson MM, Jones D, Boyett J, et al. Late mortality of long-term survivors of childhood cancer. J Clin Oncol 1997;15:2205–2213.

[9] Green DM, Zevon MA, Reese PA, et al. Factors that influence the further survival of patients who survive for five years after the diagnosis of cancer in childhood or adolescence. Med Pediatr Oncol 1994;22:91–96.

[10] Robison LL, Mertens AC. Second tumors after treatment of childhood malignancies. Hematol Oncol Clin North Am 7:401–415, 1993.

[11] Furst CJ, Lundell M, Ahlback SO et al. Breast hypoplasia following irradiation of the female breast in infancy and earlychildhood. Acta Oncol 1989;519–523.

[12] Rosenfield NS, Haller JQ, Berdon WE. Failure of development of the growing breasts after radiation therapy. Pediatr Radiol 1989;19:124–127.

[13] Rostom AY, O'Cathail S. Failure of lactation following radiotherapy for breast cancer [Letter]. Lancet 1986 Jan 18;1(8473):163–4.

[14] Leiper AD, Stanhope R, Preese MA et al. Precocious or early puberty and growth failure in girls treated for acute lymphoblastic leukemia. Horm Res 1988;30:72–76.

[15] Ogilvy-Stuart AL, Clayton PE, Shalet SM. Cranial irradiation and early puberty. J Clin Endocrinol Metab 1994;78:1282–1286.

[16] Didi M, Didcock E, Davies HA et al. High incidence of obesity in young adults after treatment of acute lymphoblastic leukemia in childhood. J Pediatr 1995;127:63–67.

[17] Oberfield SE, Soranno D, Nirenberg A et al. Age at onset of puberty following high-dose central nervous system radiation therapy. Arch Pediat Adolesc Med 1996;150:589–592.

[18] Sklar C, Mertens A, Walter A et al. Final height after treatment for childhood acute lymphoblastic leukemia: Comparison of no cranial irradiation with 1,800 and 2,400 Centigrays of cranial irradiation. J Pediatr 1993;123:59–64.

[19] Silber JH, Littman PS, Meadows AT. Stature loss following skeletal irradiation for childhood cancer. J Clin Onco1990;8:304–312.

[20] Glauser TA, Packer RJ. Cognitive deficits in long-term survivors of childhood brain tumors. Childs Nerv Syst 1991;7:2–12.

[21] Stehbens JA, Kaleih TA, Noll RB et al. CNS prophylaxis of childhood leukemia: What are the long-term neurological, neuropsycological and behavioral effects? Neuropsychol Rev 1991;2:147–176.

[22] Hoppe-Hirsch E, Renier D, Lellouch-Tubman A et al. Medulloblastoma in childhood-progressive intellectual deterioration. Childs Nerv Syst 1990;6:60–65.

[23] Ochs J, Mulher RK, Faircough D et al. Comparison of neuropsychologic function and clinical indicators of neurotoxicity in long-term survivors of childhood leukemia given cranial irradiation or parenteral methotrexate: A prospective study. J Clin Oncol 1991;9:145–151.

[24] Ash P. The influence of radiation on fertility in man. Br J Radiol 1990;53:155–158.

[25] Kreuser ED, Hetzel WD, Heit W et al. Reproductive and endocrine gonadal functions in adults following multidrug chemotherapy for acute lymphoblastic or undifferentiated leukemia. J Clin Oncol 1988;6:588–595.

[26] Koyama H, Wada T, Nishzawa Y et al. Cyclophosphamide induced ovarian failure and its therapeutic significance in patients with breast cancer. Cancer 1977;39:1403–1409.

[27] Byrne J, Fears TR, Gail MH et al. Early menopause in long term survivors of cancer during adolescence. Am J Obstet Gynecol 1992;166:788–793.

[28] Li FP, Gimbreke K, Gelber RD et al. Outcome of pregnancy in survivors of Wilms' tumor. JAMA 1987;257:216–219.

[29] Bath LE, Chambers SE, Anderson RA et al. Ovarian and uterine function following treatment for childhood cancer. 5th International Conference on Long-Term Complications of Treatment of Children and Adolescents for Cancer. Niagara-on-the-Lake, Ontario, Canada. 1998.

[30] daCunha MF, Meistrich ML, Fuller LM et al. Recovery of spermatogenesis after treatment for Hodgkin's disease: Limiting dose of MOPP chemotherapy. J Clin Oncol 1984;2:571–577.

[31] Winkel CA, Fossum GT. Current reproductive technology: consideration for the oncologist. Oncology 1993;7:40–45.

[32] Constine LS, Rubin P, Woolf PD et al. Hyperprolactinemia and hypothyroidism following cytotoxic therapy for central nervous system malignancies. J Clin Oncol 1987;5:1841–1851.

[33] Lipshultz SE, Colan SD, Gelber RD et al. Late cardiac effects of doxorubicin therapy for acute lymphoblastic leukemia in childhood. N Engl J Med 1991;324:808–814.

[34] Goorin AM, Borow KM, Goldman A et al. Congestive heart failure due to adriamycin cardiotoxicity: Its natural history in children. Cancer 1981;47:2810–2816.

[35] Steinherz LJ, Steinherz PG, Tan CT et al. Cardiac toxicity 4 to 20 years after completing anthracycline therapy. JAMA 1991;266:1672.

[36] Lipshultz SE, Colan DE. The use of echocardiography and Holter monitoring in the assessment of anthracycline-treated patients. Proceedings of the Second International Conference on Long-Term Complications of Treatment of Children and Adolescents for Cancer, Buffalo, NY, 1992.

[37] Steinherz LJ, Steinherz PG. Cardiac failure and dysrhythmias 6–19 years after anthracycline therapy: a series of 15 patients. Med Pediatr Oncol 1995;24:352–361.

[38] De Wolf D, Suys B, Maurus R et al. Dobutamine stress echocardiography min the evaluation of late anthracycline cardiotoxicity in childhood cancer survivors. Pediatr Res 1996;39:504–512.

[39] Bu'Lock FA, Mott MG, Oakhill A et al. Left ventricular diastolic function after anthracycline chemotherapy in childhood:relation with systolic function, symptoms and pathophysiology. Br Heart J 1995;73:340–350.

[40] Stewart J, Fajardo L. Radiation-induced heart disease: an update. Prog Cardivasc Dis 1984;27:173–194.

[41] Boivin JF, Hutchison GB, Lubin JH et al. Coronary artery disease mortality in patients treated for Hodgkin's disease. Cancer.1992;69:1241–1247.

[42] Hancock SL, Tucker MA, Hoppe RT. Factors affecting late mortality from heart disease after treatment of Hodgkin's disease. JAMA 1993;270:1949–1955.

[43] Hancock SL, Donaldson SS, Hoppe RT. Cardiac disease following treatment of Hodgkin's disease in children and adolescents. J Clin Oncol 1993;11:1199–1212.

[44] O'Driscoll BR, Hasleton PS, Taylor PM et al. Active lung fibrosis up to 17 years after chemotherapy with carmustine [BCNU] in childhood. N Engl J Med 1990;323:378.

[45] Samuels ML, Douglas EJ, Holoye PV et al. Large dose bleomycin therapy and pulmonary toxicity. JAMA 1976;235:1117–1120.

[46] Makipernaa A, Heino M, Laitnen L et al. Lung function following treatment of malignant tumors with surgery, radiotherapy, or cyclophosphamide in childhood. Cancer 1989;63:625–630.

[47] Van Barneveld PWC, Veenstra G, Sleifer DT et al. Changes in pulmonary function during and after bleomycin treatment in patients with testicular carcinoma. Cancer Chemother Pharmacol 1985;14:168–171.

[48] Marina NM, Greenwald CA, Fairclough DL et al. Serial pulmonary function studies in children treated for newly diagnosed Hodgkin's disease with mantle radiotherapy plus cycles of cyclophosphamide, vincristine, and procarbazine alternating with cycles of doxorubicin, bleomycin, vinblastine, and dacarbazine. Cancer 1995;75:1702–1711.

[49] Kung FH, Chauvenert AR, Ferree CR et al. Late effects on pulmonary function in children with early stage Hodgkin's disease treated with reduced dose chemoradiotherapy. Proc Am Soc Clin Oncol 1996;15:1332a.

[50] Dewit L, Anninga JK, Hoefnagel CA et al. Radiation injury in the human kidney: A prospective analysis using specific scintigraphic and biochemical endpoints. Int J Radiat Oncol Biol Phy 1990;19:977–983.

[51] Goldberg ID, Garnick MB, Bloomer WD. Urinary tract toxic\ effects of cancer therapy. J Urol 1984;132:1–6.

[52] Halperin EC, Constine LS, Tarbell NJ et al. Pediatric Radiation Oncology, Raven Press, New York; 1989.

[53] Blachley JD, Hill MB. Renal and electrolyte disturbances associated with cisplatin. Ann Intern Med 1981;95:628–632.

[54] Vogelzang NJ. Nephrotoxicity from chemotherapy: Prevention and management. Oncology 1991;5:97–112.

[55] Skinner R, Pearson AD, Price L et al. Nephrotoxicity after ifosfamide. Arch Dis Child 1990;65:732–738.

[56] Levine LA, Richie JP. Urological complications of cyclophosphamide. J Urol 1989; 141:1063–1069.

[57] Sarosy G. Ifosfamide--pharmacologic overview. Semin Oncol 1989;16:2–8.

[58] Samra Y, Hertz M, Lindner A. Urinary bladder tumors following cyclophosphamide therapy: A report of two cases with a review of the literature. Med Pediatr Oncol 1985;13:86–91.

[59] Dewit L, Ang KK, Vanderschueren E. Acute side effects and late complications after radiotherapy of localized carcinoma of the prostate. Cancer Treat Rep 1983;110:79–89.

[60] Schmipff SC. Well differentiated thyroid carcinoma: Epidemiology, etiology and treatment. Am J Med Sci 1979;278:100–114.

[61] Hudson MM, Strickland DK, Jones-Wallace C et al. Chronic hepatitis C [HCV] in childhood cancer survivors. P-16. Conference on Research Issues in Cancer Survivorship, Bethesda, MD; March 1998.

[62] Hawkins MM, Draper GJ, Kingston JE. Incidence of second primary tumors among childhood cancer survivors. Br J Cancer 1984;56:339–347.

[63] Meadows AT, Baum E, Fossati-Bellani F et al. Second malignant neoplasms in children: An update from the Late Effects Study Group. J Clin Oncol 1985;3:532–538.

[64] Zim S, Collins JM, O'Neill D et al. Inhibition of first-pass metabolism in cancer chemotherapy: Interaction of 6-mercaptopurine and allopurinol. Clin Pharmacol Ther 1983;34:810–817.

[65] Ho DJW, Frei E. Clinical pharmacology of 1-b-arabinofuranosyl cytosine. Clin Pharmacol Ther 1971;12:944–954.

[66] Hildreth NG, Shore RE, Dvortesky PM. The risk of breast cancer after irradiation of the thymus in infancy. N Engl J Med 1989;321:1281–1284.

[67] Bhatia S, Robison LL, Oberlin O et al. Breast cancer and other second neoplasms after childhood Hodgkin's disease. N Engl J Med 1996;334:745–751.

[68] Eiser C. Practitioner review: Long term consequences of childhood cancer. J Child Psychol Psychiatry 1998;39:621–633.

[69] Eiser C, Vance YH, Hill JJ. Examining the psychological consequences of surviving childhood cancer: The systematic review as a research method in pediatric psychology. J Pediatr Psychol 2000;25:449–460.

[70] Mulhern RK. Neuropsychological late effects. In: Bearison A, Mulhern R, eds. Pediatric Psychooncology. Oxford University Press, New York; 1994.

[71] Hill JM, Kornblith AB, Jones D, Freeman A, Holland JF, Glicksman AS, et al. A comparative study of the long term psychosocial functioning of childhood acute lymphoblastic leukemia survivors treated by intrathecal methotrexate with or without cranial irradiation. Cancer 1998;82:208–218.

[72] Noll RB, Bulowski WM, Davies WH, Koontz K, Kulkarni R. Adjustment in the peer system of adolescents with cancer: A twoyear study. J Pediatr Psychol 1993;18:351–364.

[73] Noll RB, MacLean WE, Whitt JK,Kaleita TA, Stehbens JA,Waskerwitz MJ, et al. Behavioral adjustment and social functioning of longterm survivors of childhood leukemia: Parent and teacher reports. J Pediatr Psychol 1997;22:827–842.

[74] Eiser C, Cool P, Grimer RJ, Carter SR, Cotter IM, Ellis AJ, et al. Quality of life following treatment for a malignant primary bone tumour around the knee. Sarcoma 1997;1:39–45.

[75] Robison LL, Nesbit ME, Sather HN, et al. Height of children successfully treated for acute lymphoblastic leukemia: A report from the late effects study committee of childrenU′ s cancer study group. Med Pediatr Oncol 1985;13:14.

[76] Lipshultz SE, Rifai N, Dalton VM, et al. The effect of dexrazoxane on myocardial injury in doxorubicin-treated children with acute lymphoblastic leukemia. N Engl J Med 2004;351:145–153.

[77] Lipshultz SE, Lipsitz SR, Sallan SE, et al. Long-term enalapril therapy for left ventricular dysfunction in doxorubicin-treated survivors of childhood cancer. J Clin Oncol 2002;20:4517– 4522.

[78] Landier W, Bhatia S, Eshelman DA, et al. Development of riskbased guidelines for pediatric cancer survivors: The Children's Oncology Group Long-Term Follow-Up Guidelines from the Children's Oncology Group Late Effects Committee and Nursing Discipline. J Clin Oncol 2004;22:4979–4990.

[79] Neglia JP, Nesbit ME Jr. Care and treatment of long-term survivors of childhood cancer. Cancer 1993;71[suppl 10]:3386–3391.

[80] Oeffinger KC, Eshelman DA, Tomlinson GE, et al. Providing primary care for long-term survivors of childhood acute lymphoblastic leukemia. J Fam Pract 2000;49:1133–1146.

[81] Schwartz CL, Constine LS. Algorithms of late effects by disease, In Schwartz CL, Hobbie W, Constine LS, et al, eds. Survivors of Childhood Cancer. Mosby, St. Louis, MO; 1994, pp. 7–19.

[82] DeLaat CA, Lampkin BC. Long-term survivors of childhood cancer: Evaluation and identification of sequelae of treatment. CA Cancer J Clin 1992;42:263–282.

[83] Lipshultz SE, Sanders SP, Goorin AM, et al. Monitoring for anthracycline cardiotoxicity. Pediatrics 1994;93:433–437.

[84] Childhood Cancer Survivorship. Improving Care and Quality of Life. Washington, DC: National Cancer Policy Board; 2003.Scottish Intercollegiate Guidelines Network [SIGN]: SIGN 50 – A guideline developers handbook. Scottish Intercollegiate Guidelines Network. Available at: www.sign.ac.uk/guidelines/fulltext/ 50/index.html.

[85] Harbour R, Miller J.Anewsystem for grading recommendations in evidence based guidelines. BMJ 2001;323:334–336.

[86] Wallace WH, Blacklay A, Eiser C, et al. Developing strategies for long term follow up of survivors of childhood cancer. BMJ 2001;323:271–274.

[87] Hudson MM, Mertens AC, Yasui Y, et al. Health status of adult long-term survivors of childhood cancer: A report from the Childhood Cancer Survivor Study. JAMA 2003;290:1583–1592.

[88] Oeffinger KC. Longitudinal risk-based health care for adult survivors of childhood cancer. Curr Probl Cancer 2003;27:143–167.

[89] Oeffinger KC, Hudson MM. Long-term complications following childhood and adolescent cancer: Foundations for providing riskbased health care for survivors. CA Cancer J Clin 2004;54:208–236.

[90] Byrne J, Lewis S, Halamek L, et al. Childhood cancer survivors' knowledge of their diagnosis and treatment. Ann Intern Med 1989;110:400–403.

[91] Mertens AC, Yasui Y, Neglia JP, et al. Late mortality experience in five-year survivors of childhood and adolescent cancer: The Childhood Cancer Survivor Study. J Clin Oncol 2001;19:3163–3172.

[92] Stevens MC, Mahler H, Parkes S. The health status of adult survivors of cancer in childhood. Eur J Cancer 1998;34:694–698.

[93] Landier W, Wallace B, Hudson MM, Long-term follow-up of pediatric cancer survivors: Education, surveillance, and screening. Pediatr Blood Cancer 2006;46:149–158.

[94] Kadan-Lottick NS, Robison LL, Gurney JG, et al. Childhood cancer survivors' knowledge about their past diagnosis and treatment: Childhood Cancer Survivor Study. JAMA 2002;287:1832–1839.

[95] Hudson MM, Tyc VL, Srivastava DK, et al. Multi-component behavioral intervention to promote health protective behaviors in childhood cancer survivors: The protect study. Med Pediatr Oncol 2002;39[2–1]:2–11.

[96] Bashore L. Childhood and adolescent cancer survivors' knowledge of their disease and effects of treatment. J Pediatr Oncol Nurs 2004;21:98–102.

[97] Caprino D, Wiley TJ, Massimo L. Childhood cancer survivors in the dark. J Clin Oncol 2004;22:2748–2750.

[98] Oeffinger KC, Hudson MM, Marina N. Knowledge, attitudes, and beliefs of physicians providing care for adult survivors of childhood cancer: A preliminary analysis [personal communication]; 2004.

[99] Taylor A, Hawkins M, Griffiths A, et al. Long-term follow-up of survivors of childhood cancer in the UK. Pediatr Blood Cancer 2004;42:161–168. Scottish Intercollegiate Guidelines Network [SIGN].

[100] Bhatia S, Anna T. Meadows, Long-term follow-up of childhood cancer survivors: Future directions for clinical care and research. Pediatr Blood Cancer 2006;46:143–148.